Health &
Happiness!

FIT FOR THE FAST TRACK

Juliette &
Nile.
(Jr. '05)

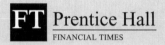

FT Prentice Hall
FINANCIAL TIMES

In an increasingly competitive world, it is quality
of thinking that gives an edge – an idea that opens new
doors, a technique that solves a problem, or an insight
that simply helps make sense of it all.

We work with leading authors in the fields of
management and finance to bring cutting-edge thinking
and best learning practice to a global market.

Under a range of leading imprints, including
Financial Times Prentice Hall, we create world-class
print publications and electronic products giving readers
knowledge and understanding which can then be
applied, whether studying or at work.

To find out more about our business and professional
products, you can visit us at www.minds.com

For other Pearson Education publications, visit
www.pearsoned-ema.com

Pearson
Education

FIT FOR
THE FAST TRACK

Surviving and Thriving in
Modern Business Life

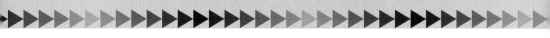

Juliette and Michael McGannon

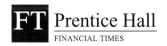

FT Prentice Hall
FINANCIAL TIMES

London · New York · Toronto · Sydney · Tokyo · Singapore · Hong Kong
Cape Town · Madrid · Paris · Amsterdam · Munich · Milan

PEARSON EDUCATION LIMITED

Head Office:
Edinburgh Gate, Harlow, Essex CM20 2JE
Tel: +44 (0)1279 623623 Fax: +44 (0)1279 431059

London Office:
128 Long Acre, London WC2E 9AN
Tel: +44 (0)207 447 2000 Fax: +44 (0)207 447 2170
Website: www.business-minds.com

First published in Great Britain in 2002

ISBN 0 273 65381 4

British Library Cataloguing in Publication Data
A CIP catalogue record for this book can be obtained from the British Library.

10 9 8 7 6 5 4 3

Designed by designdeluxe, Bath
Typeset by Pantek Arts Ltd, Maidstone, Kent
Printed and bound in Great Britain by Biddles Ltd, Guildford and King's Lynn

The Publishers' policy is to use paper manufactured from sustainable forests.

Thank you
Kevin, Jules and Seàn: for being yourselves
Gigi: merci pour les repas et les bons conseils
Nisargadatta Maharaj: for new eyes to see!

▶▶▶ *About the authors*

Juliette McGannon is the Managing Director of the McGannon Institute of Proactive Health (MIPH), France, as well as the Director of the Health Management Program (HMP) at INSEAD. She received her training in physiology and nutrition in California and specializes in fitness prescription and effective stress management. She is the innovator of the HMP, the Work–Life Balance training, the Paris Expedition, the Forest Orientation Course and SMART, a stress-management program that has been administered to over 32,000 international managers in 500 corporations. Her audio CD, *Managing Personal/Professional Balance*, has brought welcome relief to thousands of international managers worldwide. Her present projects include a multi-center research study of the impact of stress on corporate health care costs.

Dr Michael McGannon is a specialist in preventative medicine, particularly as it applies to corporate life. He holds a doctorate in medicine from Georgetown University and a post-doctoral research fellowship from Stanford University. He is also a medical journalist, writing on issues such as stress, health and fitness in international publications such as the *International Herald Tribune*, *Financial Times*, *The Business Times* (Singapore), *The European* (London) and *L'Impresa*. His first book *The Urban Warrior's Book of Solutions: Staying Healthy, Fit and Sane in the Business Jungle*, published by Financial Times Publishing, is standard issue at INSEAD and corporate management courses.

Together, Juliette and Michael McGannon have conducted the Health Management Program at business schools (including INSEAD, IMD and the Singapore Institute of Management), corporations, embassies and other organizations throughout Europe, the USA and Asia. They use many tools (computer-based learning, CD-ROM, newsletters, video and audio presentations) to provide effective insights into the means to help managers and workers manage their own survival in an environment of ever-increasing demands. They have three sons – Kevin, Jules and Seàn – and live in the French countryside near INSEAD, where they enjoy sailing, running, meditation, yoga and cooking.

►►► *Contents*

▶▶▶ *Foreword*

Since the late 1980s INSEAD has been a true pioneer in anticipating the real concerns of individual executives and multinational corporations and for finding opportunities to discuss health issues as part of our executive curriculum. Today, our Health Management Program (HMP), managed and taught by the McGannons, is a popular and valued component of all of our mainstream executive education programs.

The HMP course at INSEAD provides a desperately needed pause for reflection so that participants can take stock of their "core assets," their health and sanity, as well as the fundamental macromanagement issues that face them every day.

Managers these days, particularly at the executive level, are constantly striving to develop a real and enduring balance between their personal and professional lives. That balance begins with an awareness of their personal strengths (and weaknesses), followed by a Health Action Plan that is feasible, effective and enduring.

Presented here in this book, and based on their vast experience with many thousands of upper-caliber managers, the McGannons have designed an approach that creates the necessary awareness and provides the tools required to strike the elusive balance between work and life.

Professor Gabriel Hawawini
Dean, INSEAD
France

►►► *Acclaim for this book*

Michael and Juliette McGannon have developed unrivalled expertise in the field of executive health. Their knowledge, like this invaluable book, is based on getting to know and to really understand the pressures on more than 30,000 senior executives worldwide. *No one* knows more or how to express it better

MR. DAVID BELL, DIRECTOR OF PEOPLE, PEARSON PLC

Mike and Juliette have great insight into the stresses of modern life........This book is a must for ambitious professionals and executivess........Don't end up at age 45 with a triple heart bypass........READ THIS BOOK !!!

MR. DAVID SEDDON, SENIOR PARTNER, PwC

The well-being of our employees is the cornerstone of our success. Well-being means more to us than compensation, learning, culture ... it also includes the health of our employees. The Health Management Program described in this book has helped us in making a quantum leap to understand this ... and go for solutions.

MR. HEINZ FISCHER, EXECUTIVE VICE PRESIDENT,
DEUTSCHE BANK, GERMANY

In PricewaterhouseCoopers, we feel very fortunate to have secured the services of Michael and Juliette McGannon. Their approach to helping our people take greater responsibility for managing their own health and well-being is highly distinctive and full of simple, practical ideas. The McGannnons are a great team and they are making a *real* difference for our people.

MR. DICK WATKIN, PARTNER, PwC

...for more than the last 5 years the one element of our International Managers Development Program that has remained essentially unchanged has been the McGannons' Health Management Program described herein. Not only has it received the *highest* scores in the feedback from participants, but it has had a lasting positive impact on the hundreds of managers who have experienced the Program. *If you are really serious about your people being your most valuable asset then tell them to read this book to help them to look after their health!*

MR. PATRICK THOMAS, PRESIDENT,
HUNTSMAN SPECIALTY CHEMICALS, BELGIUM

No matter how wealthy you may be, nor how successful, you have nothing unless you have your health and you enjoy your life. I have had the privilege of knowing and working with the McGannons, Michael and Juliette, since 1985. No one is more qualified, nor are there any better more straightforward principles, than those enunciated by them in these pages and at their Institute of Health. *If your health and sanity mean anything to you, this book is a must read.*

MR. RON CLARKE, RECORD HOLDER (19 WORLD, 35 AUSTRALIAN) IN
LONG-DISTANCE RUNNING, CEO, INTERPACIFIC RESORTS AUSTRALIA

On reflection, one always finds some events which change people's behaviour and life. For me the Health Management Program (HMP) was one such event. Mike and Juliette, with their lucid communication, brought to life a strong sense of the urgent need to change my diet and life style. I have been practising some of the methods recommended by Mike and Juliette; this has indeed made a difference to both my physical and mental health. I would strongly advocate that all managers working for me read this book and attend this programme. I am sure they too will benefit.

MR. ANNOOTTAM GHOSH, CHIEF EXECUTIVE,
PERFORMANCE CHEMICALS, ICI INDIA LTD

Roughly 100 of my Taiwanese colleagues volunteered to take the Health Management Program. Their reactions ranged from positive to ecstatic. They were impressed by the enthusiasm which Michael and Juliette brought to the health of each participant. Unlike many professionals in medicine, Michael and Juliette radiate health. Read the book, follow the Progam, and you too can be in the pink.

MR. MICHAEL WHITEHEAD, COUNTRY MANAGER, CATHAY PACIFIC, JAPAN

McGannon's HMP and course text have been one of the most enlightening and impact learning experiences in my life. It has really affected the way I take responsibility of a very challenging life style while ensuring long-term balance, energy and health. McGannon's approach to health management is full of common sense and is actually doable. With simple and small twists in my habits I found myself with higher levels of energy, health and ability to enjoy both life and business challenges. Today, after more than four years since I went through McGannon's HMP, I continue to practice what I learnt. It is now so naturally integrated in my life style that it does not require any heroic decision to keep it. Virtually every single manager that went through the program expressed very similar insights on the value and real impact it had on their lives, their families and their businesses.

MR. JOSÉ CONEJOS, SENIOR MANAGER, HEWLETT-PACKARD

The Health Management Program described within, as conducted by Michael and Juliette, is *truly remarkable*. What makes it so special is the passion and commitment they bring to the program. It is a MUST DO program text for any one who wants to stay healthy and fit. The best part is that you love every moment of it.

MS. NIRA ANAND, HEAD, HUMAN RESOURCES,
THE WORLD BANK, NEW DELHI

Most programs fail because they take a rigorous approach to fitness. The twenty-minute HMP program can be done ANYTIME, ANYWHERE. Twenty minutes a day works! It has been wonderful to see how much the people in our company, who have adopted these principles, have benefited. Health is one of our most important assets and this program is the most important gift that you can give to others to encourage them achieve that goal. *A must do!*

MR. PAUL RODE, CHIEF FINANCIAL OFFICER,
NORTH AMERICA, MOTOROLA CORPORATION

Juliette and Michael McGannon are opening up a whole new way for us harried business folks to look at who we are and what we do with our lives. In this book, they are rekindling the flame of self-discovery.

MR. SUNIL KISHORE, HEAD, HUMAN RESOURCES, THE OBEROI GROUP

▶▶▶ *A Personal Note from the Authors*

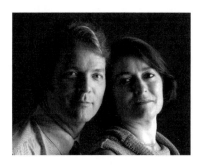

Dear Reader

There is a particularly nasty myth out there in the business community that getting and staying in the shape necessary to stay competitive takes a lot of time, pain, and effort. Just not so! Our hands-on experience with more than 30,000 managers from over 400 corporations and the prevalent scientific data both strongly support the idea that staying healthy and sane is more a question of strategic choices, not brute work or overexertion. After all, on their deathbed, no one wishes they had spent more time at the office!

Our purpose in writing this work is not to propose or endorse specific models of health, but to direct the modern manager towards those tools (mental and physical) that will empower them to achieve optimal personal and professional balance. Towards this end, we have married together the French *savoir vivre* with American science tradition to develop a complete set of highly effective and feasible health tools to help weave a little hygiene into the lives of managers worldwide.

We are very grateful to the managers with whom we have had the privilege of working at INSEAD, since leaving Stanford University in 1988. It is through the careful listening to them that we were able to innovate the healthy program contained in this book.

Lastly, we hope that the advice and tools contained herein are of use to you in striking that elusive balance between the two aspects of life that give it most meaning and pleasure: work and family.

Bon courage and enjoy!

Juliette and Michael McGannon
Directors, Health Management Program, INSEAD
Co-founders, MIPH

INTRODUCTION

MODELS OF HEALTH

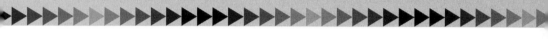

Life moves so much more rapidly now than it ever did before ... the huge acceleration in the rate of growth of facts, of knowledge, of techniques, of inventions, of advances in technology ... We need a different type of human being ... who is comfortable with change, who enjoys change, who is able to improvise, who is able to face with confidence, strength and courage a situation of which he has absolutely no forewarning ... the society which can turn out such people will survive; the societies that cannot turn out such people will die.

ABRAHAM MASLOW, 1950s

Truly a Lazy Person's Program!

Our research involving more than 30,000 international managers has proven without a shred of doubt that when it comes to surviving and even thriving in the fast track of international business, compensation (*not* deprivation) works best. Through scientifically proven tools of compensation, our research has found that most managers can dramatically improve their health, fitness and sanity in only 20 minutes per day.[1] In terms of efficacy, a lot of sweating and suffering is even counterproductive!

Various Work–Life Models

The Disease–Care Model

In today's global fast-track economies, having a management that is hardy and resistant to the stresses of the profession is not a luxury, it is a *competitive necessity*. International business life is fraught with inherent hazards: long hours of highly stressful work, separation from our loved ones, long periods of physical inactivity, rich nutrition, excessive alcohol … and the consequences appear every day in the obituary columns.

The disease–care model is so called because that is where we, the members of the medical community, spend most of our efforts and time: caring for diseases, *not* preserving health. The classic approach to balance between work and life by international managers is shown in Fig I.1.

Everything in our lives is defined and justified in terms of work. It is a rather stoic model: a consistently *extreme* approach to work (where even weekends are fair game), to physical exercise (nothing or too much, but generally, sedentary), to nutrition (low-fiber, highly refined sugars and

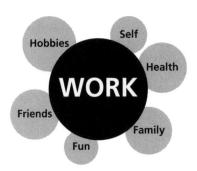

FIGURE I.1 *Non-sustainable work–life imbalance*

processed foods, and, perhaps, eating a very low fat diet). This model – the dominant model in places like the USA, UK, northern Europe and parts of Asia – stresses wealth at the expense of health: "No pain, no gain," "Just do it!".

As a result, it is estimated that more than 50% of Americans are currently obese (versus 24% in 1960, 35% in 1990,[2] and an estimated 75% by 2020, if current trends continue). When the 20th century began, CVD[3] was responsible for less than 10% of all deaths worldwide. Only 100 years later, that figure has skyrocketed to over 50% in the industrialized countries and nearly 30% in the still developing world. The work–life imbalance shown in Fig. I.1 is a very important part of the reason. The results for the business community are disastrous: managers are routinely unable to fulfill their functions adequately because of increased incidence of heart disease, diabetes, strokes, depression, premature cancers, stress-related diseases, obesity and chronic fatigue. Must the price for success be so exorbitant? The answer, after 14 years of research involving more than 30,000 managers from 40 different countries, is clearly "no."

Our research indicates a solid work–life balance is not only possible but feasible!

Vitality Model

What we have been developing with the many thousands of international managers with whom we work is an alternative approach to the work–life balance, shown in Fig. I.2.

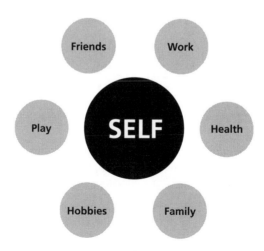

FIGURE I.2 *Sustainable work–life balance*

The **vitality model** approach to health and vitality is radically different to the unsustainable approach because of its strong emphasis on the preservation of what we call our core assets: our health and sanity. This involves the use of appropriate stress management techniques, optimized nutrition and a customized physical activity program. This more sustainable model of work–life balance emphasizes the health, *then* wealth concept. The main focus of health care is to *reinforce the defenses of the body* (the terrain within – the *internal milieu* – as discussed by Louis Pasteur and Claude Bernard).

The result is a more hardy, pleasure-oriented, spontaneous approach to activity (leisure walks during the weekend with family, participation in team sports), education through culture, little or no refined or junk foods, very little refined sugar and a more balanced attitude towards fat consumption. Corporations[4] and cultures that provide an opportunity for their members to strike a balance between work and private life seem to have the best health and longest longevity, two critical components of vitality.[5]

Now compare the various indicators for the cultures that embrace a more sustainable work–life balance (see Table I.1).

TABLE I.1 *Indicators for a sustainable work–life balance*

Country	CVD (rate per 100,000)	Diabetes (rate per 100,000)	Life expectancy at birth (world rank)	Overall health care[6] (world rank)
France	578.4	23	73.1 (3rd)	1
Japan	465.4	19.8	74.5 (1st)	10
UK	871.5	22	71.7 (14th)	18
USA[7]	698.6	47.8	70 (24th)	37

Source: World Health Organization

Meet Mr Timebomb

Since 1988, while based at INSEAD, we have been carrying out in-depth research involving more than 30,000 international managers from over 40 countries to test which model of health works best. The challenge was to develop an eclectic model of health that would be effective in delaying aging and avoiding some of the health issues that plague the business community: heart disease, diabetes, depression, stress-related problems, low stamina and obesity and related blood tests (TG, TC, low HDL). What follows is a compilation of the health check-ups of more than 30,000 managers. Take out your latest check-up and see how you would stack up against Mr Timebomb – a typical example of one of the world's premier fast trackers.

Before

- **Overview of Life:** A normal 42-year-old man, with modern ambitions who works for a telecom concern and enjoys his work. Social state: worries often, feels anxious for no real reason. Family history: prostate cancer, diabetes and hypertension.
- **Main complaints:** He has noticed over the past three years that he has begun snorting while laughing and snoring while sleeping. He is also experiencing chronic back pain, extended bouts of fatigue and sharp pain in foot joints.
- **Medical exam:**
  - **Blood pressure (BP)** = 165/95 (normal < 135/85).
  - **Heart fitness** = 150 beats (normal < 90 beats).
  - **Body fat (BF)** = 30% (normal < 20%).
  - **Blood work:**
    - **total cholesterol (TC)** = 2.65 grams/liter[8] (normal < 2.00 g/l) (the average cholesterol level of a heart attack victim is about 2.4 g/l);
    - **HDL (the "good") cholesterol** = 0.35 g/l (normal > 0.50 g/l);
    - **blood triglycerides (TGs = blood fats)** = 2.40 g/l (normal < 1.40 g/l);
    - **blood sugar** = 1.60 g/l (normal < 1.10 g/l).
  - **Health age.**[9] 65.7.
  - **Very high risk** of the following medical problems:
    - heart attack
    - strokes
    - diabetes
    - depression, isolation, withdrawal …
    - gout.

After six months of following the advice in this book

- **Overview of life:** The same 42-year-old man without any specific complaints or symptoms. He reports ample energy to cope with family, work and self.
- **Medical exam:**
  - **Blood pressure** = 120/70.
  - **Heart fitness** = 83 beats.

- **Body fat** = 20%.
- **Blood work** (all normalized):
  - **total cholesterol** = 1.83 g/l;
  - **HDL cholesterol** = 0.68 g/l;
  - **blood triglycerides** = 0.75 g/l;
  - **blood sugar** = 0.79 g/l.
- **Health age:** 39.3.
- **Low risk** of disease, depression and low-fatigue states.

Model for the New Millennium

When developing the model of the relationship between the *internal milieu* (the internal space or the immune network) and the *external milieu* (the invading microbes), Louis Pasteur, the father of modern microbiology, emphasized the importance of the internal terrain in maintaining proper health. He is quoted as saying:

So often I see weakened or stressed human beings who no longer have sufficient internal hardiness to resist the invasion of microscopic organisms.

This model of the body and mind would suggest that, although there are certain aspects of life we cannot control, one aspect we can control is our internal defenses, our state of preparedness: the state of our internal terrain, our hardiness. We can make ourselves more resistant to potentially harmful events by upgrading not just the body's defenses (through physical activity and pure nutrition) but also the mind's defenses (the way we perceive the world).

The vitality model of the new millennium, combining salient aspects of all the above models, seems to work best. This combines the nutrition and internal resistance of the southern European model (including wine drinking), the work hard and play hard life ethic of the Anglo-American model, and the mind control aspects of the Asian model into a model that emphasizes vitality (from the Latin *vita* = life) – physical fitness, positive attitude, the life force, the chi, the Brahman, the soul – as its central concept. Such a strategy works best for maintaining vitality and health and is far more in alignment with our primitive origins.

Looking at Fig. I.3, consider the following:

- At what age would I like to peak, physically? Mentally?
  Answer: when you want.

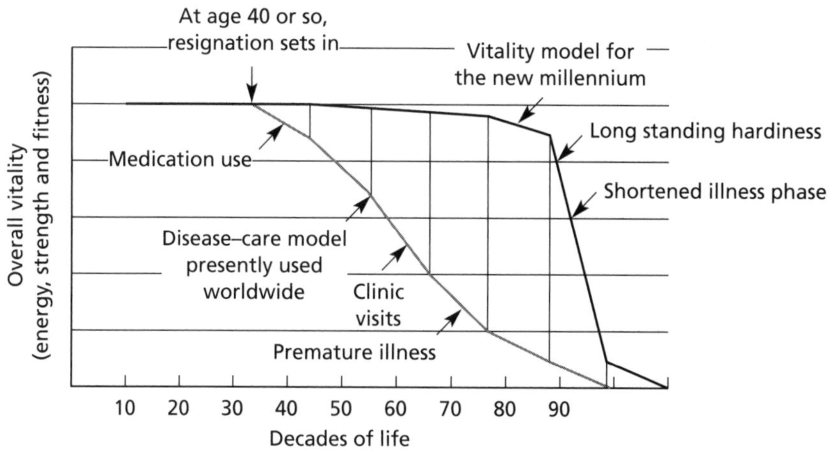

FIGURE 1.3 *Vitality and age*

■ What shape would I like to be in when (if) I retire?   *Answer:* the condition you want.

■ Could it be that disease begins in the mind, with attitude? *Answer:* yes.

■ Could 40 years of working life become a mere warm-up for life's other adventures?   *Answer:* possibly.

This book

As already discussed, the purpose of this book is not to focus on individual models of health but rather to provide you, the reader, with those mental and physical tools you require to ensure that you can survive and thrive in modern business life. To this end, the text has been broadly divided into the following sections (the 6Ws to peak personal professional balance):

■ A quantifiable enquiry into the physiologic upgrading of the **body** (Walking, Water, Wine, and Workout). (Chapters 1–4.)

■ An enquiry, though less amenable to scientific quantification, devoted to the upgrading of the **mind** (Worrying effectively and Wind), using psychology as the scalpel of choice. (Chapters 5 and 6.)

Our research indicates one final reality: a solid work–life balance is possible!

Frequently Asked Questions[10]

Heart Disease and Culture

Q How are different cultures faring in the battle against **heart disease**?

Europe

■ Within Europe, in two recent prospective studies, men and women with the highest intake of Vitamin E (from supplements) had a *40% decrease in heart-attack risk*.

■ Studies in France confirm that the "Americanization" of Europe has established a beachhead in France: the rate of obesity among children increased by 17% between 1980 and 1990 and extreme obesity has increased by 28%, due to reduced physical activity, more junk foods and less regular hot meals.

■ Premature (< 60 years) death rates from cardiovascular disease range from 40.5/100,000 in France to 245/100,000 in Latvia.

Asia

■ Health is often seen as a price tag for wealth.

■ Asians, because of their smaller frames, develop obesity-related diseases at lower obesity levels than Europeans.

■ In Taiwan, the number of deaths from diabetes (80% of which cases are due to obesity) has tripled since 1985.

■ In Singapore, cases of diabetes have doubled since 1992.

India

■ In the year 2001, there are approximately 22 million diabetics in India. According to the World Health Organization (WHO), by the year 2025 there will be 57 million, an increase of 260% in just 25 years!

■ The All Indian Institute of Medical Sciences observed that the proportion of patients entering tertiary care facilities with coronary artery disease (CAD) has risen over the past 30 years from 4 to 33%.

■ In a survey in progress in urban Delhi, measuring high blood pressure (> 140/90), a prevalence of 17.4% has been observed in persons between 35 and 64 years of age, while blood pressure (> 160/90) ranges from 4.3 to 12.1%.

Eastern Mediterranean

■ The proportion of deaths from cardiovascular disease ranges from 25 to 45%.

■ Among Saudi Arabians aged 18–74, 52% of males and 65% of females are obese.

China

■ Death rates from cardiovascular disease have shown an increase from 86/100,000 in 1957 to 214/100,000 in 1990.

■ Adult smokers: 61% males, 7% females.

■ There are possibly as many as 60 million hypertensives. Stroke has four times the incidence of heart attacks.

■ There are between one million and one and a half million strokes every year.

■ Taken all together, cardiovascular disease claims about 2.5 million lives (about 30% of all deaths).

The Americas

■ Obesity data – one statistic suffices: 24% overfat in 1960, 35% in 1990. The reasons:

  – According to the US Department of Agriculture, the top 10 sources of calories in the average American diet are (with Glycemic Index): cola, white bread (GI = 101), doughnut (GI = 108), table sugar (GI = 101), white flour (GI = 101), processed cheese, beef, 2% milk (GI = 48).

  – Almost 50% of American youth (12–21 years of age) get no regular vigorous activity and the proportion of high school students (13–17 years of age) getting daily physical education at school dropped from 42% in 1991 to 25% in 1995.

  – The direct and indirect costs for heart attacks and strokes in the USA alone for one year amount to US$ 326.6 billion.

Africa

■ Cigarette consumption has increased in Africa by 40% in the last two decades.

■ Cardiovascular disease ranges from 20 to 45% and this figure is changing rapidly for the worst, particularly in northern African countries.

Blood Pressure/Heart Disease

Q What is more important for heart risk: **systolic** (SBP) or **diastolic** blood pressure (DBP)?

■ Of the two figures, SBP is a better predictor of heart attacks, strokes and heart failure. However, it must be understood that blood pressure is defined in stages: normal, high-normal, and hypertensive. Regardless of age, the ideal SBP is < 130 over < 85 (diastolic), according to the Joint National Committee on Prevention, Detection, Evaluation and Treatment of High Blood Pressure (JNC-VI). Table I.2 gives the guidelines for the JNC-VI.

TABLE I.2 *JNC-VI criteria for blood pressure*

Category	SBP		DBP
Optimal	< 120	*and*	< 80
Normal	< 130	*and*	< 85
High-normal	130–139	*or*	85–89
Hypertension:			
Stage 1	140–159	*or*	90–99
Stage 2	160–179	*or*	100–109
Stage 3	> 180	*or*	> 110

Q What is a **heart attack**?

■ A poor name for a compromised blood supply to the **heart muscle**. The heart arteries are blocked by both thickened blood and plaque.

Q How would I know if I were at **high risk** of a heart attack or stroke?

■ You have increased risk of a heart attack or stroke if you fall into any of the following categories:

 – you smoke cigarettes;

 – your blood pressure is regularly above 140/90;

 – you are physically inactive;

 – your stress is not compensated;

 – you have poorly controlled diabetes;

 – you are depressed.

Q What is a **stroke**?

■ A poor name for a compromised blood supply to the **brain**. Most (90%) strokes are due to a blockage by a clot of blood (ischemic stroke), while, thankfully, only 10% bleed (hemorrhagic stroke). Green leafy vegetables and citrus fruits provide some protection against strokes.[11]

Q At what **age** does heart disease begin?

■ New studies of teenagers carried out by the American Heart Association have established that, while symptoms of heart disease begin in middle age or older, the process of arteriosclerosis begins in the teens.

Q Can the companionship offered by **pets** affect my blood pressure (BP)?

■ Researchers studied 48 stockbrokers (male and female) who were using medication to control BP. Those with a pet had half the high BP associated with stress experienced by those without companionship. Proof again that isolation hurts health.

Q What is the relationship between **salt** and blood pressure?

■ The newest data on patients with BP > 120/80 indicate that systolic BP declined progressively as salt intake decreased. A major obstacle to lowering salt intake is fast and processed foods.[12]

Diabetes

Q Is there a link between diabetes and **coronary artery diseases (CAD)**?

■ Diabetes increases the risk, prevalence, severity and virulence of CAD. Type II diabetes carries a two- to four-fold increase in the risk for CAD (American Heart Association).

■ Elevated insulin levels are associated with thickened blood and thrombosis.[13]

Q If Type II (adult onset) diabetics already have a relative lack of insulin, why are they at **increased risk of heart disease**?

■ Because these Type II diabetics (comprising 90–95% of the world's diabetics) eventually develop insulin resistance, so that the cells of the body stop responding to the insulin instructions to let the sugar into the cell. Result: both sugar and insulin rise in the blood as the pancreas tries in vain to force the sugar into the cell, until the pancreas tires out and stops producing insulin altogether. At this point, the disease reaches a crisis point and the patient now requires insulin by injections.

Notes

1 See Epilogue to see the scientifically proven implementation of the 100 Timebomb cases.

2 *Morbidity/Mortality Weekly Review*, 1999; 48: 649–56.

3 Cardiovascular diseases (CVD) include: high blood pressure, coronary artery disease (CAD), strokes, arrythmias, congestive heart failure and rheumatic and other valvular heart disease. By 2025, CVD will be responsible for at least 25 million deaths per year and coronary artery disease (CAD) will surpass infectious diseases as the number-one cause of death and disease, worldwide.

4 Virtually all the corporations for whom we have set up in-house health seminars to assist their managers to confront the inherent health dangers facing the international business community (including such stars as PwC, ICI, HP, MaxIndia, Andersen, Cathay Pacific, Motorola, Uniqema, Henkel, Standard Chartered Bank, Dragon Air) have shown tangible, as well as subjective, benefits by striving for a healthier more balanced work environment.

5 The Japanese have the greatest longevity due to: (1) lots of walking (2) a very pure nutrition (based on raw fish and little sugar or saturated fat) resulting in very low rate of coronary artery disease, and (3) very strong traditional ties that counterbalance the inordinately long work hours.

6 Positions 3, 4, 5 are occupied by three other Mediterranean countries: San Marino, Andorra and Malta, respectively. The World Health Organization (WHO) has conducted an unprecedented analysis of the world's health care systems, using performance indicators to measure the health systems of the 191 member states. See *The World Health Report 2000 – Health Systems: Improving Performance*.

7 Reasons for this poor ranking, despite spending the highest proportionally on disease care than any other country, include: (1) high rate of coronary artery disease (CAD) (2) high tobacco-related deaths (3) high sugar intake resulting in high obesity levels, and (4) low physical activity.

8 Conversion factors for laboratory values:
   – for the cholesterol family (TC, HDL, LDL): from mmol/l to grams/liter, *divide* by 2.6 (5.2 mmol/l 2.6 = 2.0 g/l);
   – for the TGs: from mmol/l to grams/liter, *divide* by 1.17 (2.9 mmol/l / 1.17 = 2.5 g/l);
   – for the fasting blood sugar (glucose): from mmol/l to grams/liter, *divide* by 5.5 (8.3 mmol/l / 5.5 = 1.5 g/l).

9 A statistical analysis, using health data from the World Health Organization, local government health agencies and insurance companies, demonstrating the overall impact of lifestyle on longevity. As seen here with the illustrative case, a Health Age in excess of the Actual Age would indicate an accelerated aging process due to inactivity, obesity, fat abnormalities and so on.

10 The FAQs presented here are actual queries that have arisen in one form or another in our seminars with more than 30,000 managers, either at INSEAD or within corporations, since 1988.

11 *Journal of the American Medical Association*, 1999; 282: 1233–9.

12 *New England Journal of Medicine*, 2001; Jan 4; 344: 3–10.

13 *Journal of the American Medical Association*, 2000; 283: 221–8.

CHAPTER ONE

WALKING

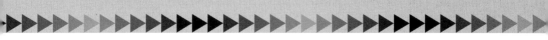

Why jog, when walking has been proven to be the easiest and most efficient way to lose body fat?

Using the advice contained in this chapter, Mr Timebomb could take care of the following health issues:

- high blood pressure
- high body fat/waist-to-hip ratio
- high cholesterol
- high blood triglycerides
- low HDL (good) cholesterol
- low stamina
- high blood sugar.

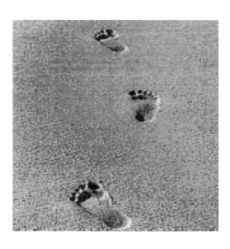

Introduction

Walking has a long and glorious history of healing not just our arteries, but our hearts and souls as well. It is also the single most effective and feasible exercise to mobilize body fat.

Did you realize that the weight-loss industry worldwide has the dubious distinction of being the only human enterprise that dedicates billions of dollars to losing something but which is largely ineffective?

What is Body Fat?

Figure 1.1 shows the different compartments into which body fat can be broken down.

You have heard the expression "You are what you eat." That is most certainly the case when we discuss body fat. But as well as being the part of the body on which the multibillion-dollar weight-loss industry focusses its attention, body fat is essential to health as an insulator, shock absorber and energy source during famine.

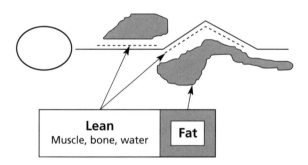

FIG. 1.1 *The body-fat compartments*

How to Measure Body Fat

There are essentially three ways to measure body fat:

1 *Hydrostatic weighing:* fat has a specific gravity (density) less than that of water and of lean mass (muscle and bone). Hence, fat floats on water. Therefore, to measure the bouyancy effect of body fat, you

weigh yourself on dry land and then under water. A research tool with excellent accuracy, but highly impractical.

2 *Fat calipers:* notorious inaccuracy and requires expensive calipers and software to assess.

3 *Circumference:* based on the hydrostatic weighing procedure (accurate) and very practical (just a tape measure in centimeters required). Here are the formulae for measuring your body fat, which can then be used to correlate your overall health (blood pressure, heart disease), stamina levels and laboratory tests (especially total cholesterol, triglycerides and blood sugar):

Men: ((waist (cm) / 2.54 – 3) + (hips (cm) / 2.54 + 1) – (forearm (cm) / 2.54) X 3) – 19 = _____ BF %

Women: ((waist (cm) / 2.54 – 6) + (thigh (cm) / 2.54 + 4) – (calf (cm) / 2.54) X 1.5) – 21 = _____ BF %

Excessive body fat is defined as > 20% for men and > 23% for women. High body fat, especially when the circumference of the waist divided by the circumference of the hips is > 0.95, is associated with the following:

■ high blood pressure[1] (body fat is a very vascular tissue: the more body fat one has, the harder the heart has to work)

■ high blood triglycerides (TGs)

■ heart attacks and premature death

■ diabetes

■ disability in older age.[2]

Getting Rid of the Body Fat You Already Have

Understanding and Engineering Your Metabolic Rate

Nearly everyone is familiar with the concept of metabolic rate. Metabolic rate is *the* keystone to body fat control.

The metabolic rate is defined as the energy/heat (calories) expended by the body in a set time frame. The unit employed is calories/day. The higher the metabolic rate, the less body fat there is present. Normally, the metabolic rate is high in the morning, as you are getting your day going, so it makes great sense to adhere to the age-old maxim:

> Eat a breakfast of kings
> Eat a lunch of princes
> Eat a dinner of paupers.

The lifestyle factors that increase the metabolic rate are as follows:

1 *Physical activity:* the more spontaneously active you are, the less need there is for working out in gyms. Walking for 15 minutes at one left-right (L/R) cycle per second (3.5 miles or 5 km/hour) will generate approximately 90 calories of heat.

2 *Food:* incoming calories tell the body that it can continue burning calories – this is called the Thermic Effect of Food (TEF). TEF can be up to 10% of total calories. In other words, if your heaviest meal consists of 1,000 calories, your body requires 100 calories just to process the food. The TEF peaks at 60 minutes after the meal.

Window of opportunity

Taken together, activity and TEF have a *synergistic* effect. That is, for every one minute spent on low-grade[3] activity within the 30–60 minutes after a meal, your body accelerates the metabolic rate for 3 minutes! Practically speaking, if you walk 15 minutes after your meal, once you are back, you increase your calorie burning for 45 minutes. That's why we call this a Lazy Person's Program: how little you can do to gain the maximal return!

We call this a Lazy Person's Program: how little you can do to gain the maximal return!

So, every day immediately after (within 30 minutes) your heaviest meal, do a metabolic walk, at a rate of one L/R cycle per second (3.5 miles/hour or 5 km/hour). The meal (the meal has a TEF = 100 calories) + the brisk walk (equivalent to 90 calories[4]) will result in a loss of up to 7.7 kilograms (17 pounds) from your fat compartment per year! In addition, this strategy is accompanied by a 30% decrease in mortality due to heart disease, stroke, diabetes and other obesity-related issue.[5]

The Biophysiology of Walking

Looking at Fig. 1.2, several undisputed facts will become clear.

Fact 1: Oxygen (O_2) is the key

Look at the structure and oxygen content of the two main fuels of the body: fats and carbohydrates (carbohydrates are the components of the sugar family). The generic structure of fat is $C_{16}H_{32}O_2$ and the generic structure of sugar is $C_6H_{12}O_6$. Note the ratio between carbon and oxygen for each fuel. Which fuel contains more oxygen? Answer: carbohydrates (sugars).

Fact 2: The intensity of the activity determines the fuel selected

Since the whole point of food is to provide calories and oxygen to the body, the body chooses the fuel it will need on the basis of how much oxygen is required. Two illustrative examples:

1 *High-intensity exercises (squash, sprinting, marathon running)* require tremendous amounts of O_2 in order to meet the demands of the muscles (more than the heart and lungs can offer) and, therefore, choose carbohydrate as a major fuel source (80%). It has been

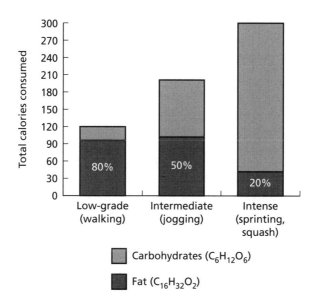

FIGURE 1.2 *How the body synchronizes fuel with activity*

repeatedly demonstrated that as the exercise intensity increases (above 50% of CO_2 max), there exists an absolute requirement that if the bulk of energy needs are not met by high-O_2 carbohydrates, the exercise must stop or reduce intensity. That is precisely why marathon runners do what is called "carbo-loading" prior to the race to load the liver and muscles with stored carbohydrates (glycogen). Working out harder may actually leave you fatter!

2 *Low-intensity exercise (walking)* requires much less O_2 and, therefore, uses body fat as a predominant (80%) source of fuel which actually increases further as the exercise (walking) continues. As the exercise becomes increasingly intense (from a walk to a jog) and the oxygen needs rise, the body switches from a predominant fat source to a mixture of fat-carbohydrate (glycogen).

Fact 3: There is an optimal time for metabolic walking

The best time for metabolic walking is after your largest meal. Lunchtime is the best from a practical standpoint, as you need not leave the home at night.

But let's face it – metabolic walking is all right for those cool days along the Hudson or Thames Rivers, but a power walk at noon in Singapore or Kuala Lumpur or in December in Geneva is tough going. Think creatively!

If the pollution gets too much or the heat and humidity starts soaring, take to the biggest walk-in refrigerators around: the malls. For those of you in hot climates, the first step is to find the closest shopping mall that is climate controlled. Check the hours during which the mall is opened and not so crowded. Start on the ground floor and walk briskly (taking short strides and swinging arms) from one end of the mall to the other. Jog up the stairways or escalator and repeat on the next floor until you reach the top. Now turn around and come down.

Important health note: in a recent study,[6] it was shown that elderly men (aged 71–93) who walked 2 miles (3 km) a day had *half* the heart attack rate of men who walked 0.25 miles (0.50 km) a day, with the overall heart attack rate dropping 15% for each half mile (about 1 km) walked.

In summary, recent research has shown that metabolic walking has numerous benefits:

1 *Disease prevention:* people who walk up to 5 hours weekly are half as likely to have elevated body fat and cholesterol. In practice, metabolic walking for 30 minutes per day several days a week can dramatically reduce the risk (in men and women) for heart disease and cardiac

death by 30% because of normalization of blood pressure, body fat, triglycerides and an increase in the HDL ("good") cholesterol.

2 *Increasing bone mass:* metabolic walking is a weight-bearing exercise (swimming is not). As such, metabolic walking increases bone mass by laying down new bone, thereby slowing the onset and severity of osteoporosis.

3 *Increases in stamina:* instead of a coffee break, go for an "energy break": metabolic walking and two glasses of water or fresh fruit juice.

4 *Better mental fitness:* a natural result of communing with Nature, conversing with friends and feeling the silence.

5 *High accessibility:* no requirement for sportswear and easy access for beginners make this "everybody's sport." Best of all, it doesn't cost any money!

Preventing Body Fat

What Works Best: a Low-Sugar or Low-Fat Diet?

There is an ongoing battle in the medical community between low-fat and low-sugar diets. When it comes to losing body fat, it means that there are definite cultural differences reflected in attitudes towards life, health and nutrition:

1 *Low-sugar diet:* involves less refined junk foods, compensating occasional excesses with low-grade aerobic activity (walking) and eating more balanced foods (the preferred first approach for our managers).

2 *Low-fat diet:* includes calorie counting and deprivation. According to a 1997 study[7] low-fat diets do not affect body weight and actually *lowered* total cholesterol and HDL (good cholesterol) proportionally. Moreover, it has been amply demonstrated that calorie restriction results in lower activity and metabolism levels, very possibly a risk factor for cancers.

Our own research[8] since 1988 shows that a full 80% of our 30,000 participants respond superbly to a low-sugar regimen to control body fat, cholesterol, triglycerides (TGs), HDL and kindred issues, such as heart disease, strokes, diabetes, obesity, cancers and low energy states. During that time, we have had the opportunity of studying these respective strategies independently with a predictable result: the EuroAsian model not only seems to work better and faster, but participants find it easier to adapt to their specific culture and, therefore, to comply with.

Therefore, following a sensible and scientific approach for people with excessive body fat and related issues (low stamina, high cholesterol, high triglycerides, low HDL and diabetes), we would suggest a scientifically-proven three-tier strategy. Start with:

1 **A low-sugar strategy (LSS)**: that is, low Glycemic Index foods, discussed below. Check the results (body fat and laboratory results) after three months: suboptimal or no change?

2 **A low-fat strategy[9] (LFS)**: check the results (body fat and laboratory results): suboptimal or no change?

3 **A low-cholesterol strategy[10] (LCS)**: chances are excellent that you will never need to go this far.

Insulin

The Key Player to Control Body Fat

Understand insulin and you understand health Understand insulin and you understand health. Not to understand insulin is to bypass the simplest and most effective way to optimize not just body fat, but overall health, vitality and longevity. What are the physiologic actions of insulin? Five minutes of committing to memory these actions could translate into many years of health.

In **normal situations**, insulin:

■ is secreted by the pancreas. Its $T \frac{1}{2}$ (the time required to clear $\frac{1}{2}$ the original amount) = 7–15 minutes;

■ transports sugar, its main stimulus, into the cells of the body where the sugar can be used for energy;

■ stores sugar, protein and fat in fat cells as triglycerides and inhibits fat breakdown;

■ increases in response to fructose and proteins only in the presence of already elevated blood sugar levels (such as in obese people).

In **abnormal situations**, when provoked by excessive sugar intake, elevated insulin:

vitality, let's identify the foods that make insulin surge (see Table 1.1). As sugar is the main stimulus for insulin secretion, the greater the blood sugar rise, the greater the insulin surge. So, high GI foods promote high body fat, high TGs, high LDL and low HDL cholesterol levels – all important components for heart disease.

The Glycemic Index provides the key to achieving low insulin levels

Looking at Table 1.1, therefore, if you are fairly sedentary and *not* about to run a marathon, these are the types of fuel you should avoid as they will stimulate insulin and store body fat.

TABLE 1.1 *High Glycemic Index foods*

High Glycemic Index foods	GI
Maltose (beer sugar)	150
Dates	146
Glucose (sugar, refined)	137
French baguette, Lucozade	136
Wheat bread (gluten free)	129
White rice (instant boiled)	128
Honey	126
Raggi	123
Potato (baked, instant, microwaved)	117–121
Cornflakes	119
Cooked carrots, Rice Krispies	117
Pretzels	116
Tapioca (boiled with milk)	115
Jelly beans	114
Morning coffee cookies	113
Rice cakes, Jowar, Cocopops	110
Waffles, Total cereal	109
Doughnut	108
French fries (chips)	107
Cheerios, bread stuffing	106
Corn chips	105
White bagel, watermelon	103
White bread, millet, maize meal porridge	101
Lifesavers, wheat biscuits, Crème of Wheat	100
Wheat bread, wholemeal flour	100
Skittles, corn meal	98
Taco shells, Fanta, Varagu	97
Croissant, Grapenuts, stone wheat thins	96
Gnocchi, angel food cake	95
Canned pea soup, pineapple, NutriGrain, Life	94

TABLE 1.1 *continued*

High Glycemic Index foods	GI
Couscous, steamed potato, cantaloupe	93
Black bean soup, rye bread	92
Beets, raisins	91
Maize chapati, Shredded Wheat, muffins	89
Muesli bar, ice cream	87
Split pea soup, cheese pizza	86
Vermicelli (fine noodles). Take out honey	83
Apricots (fresh), bajra (millet)	82
Sultana, mango, muesli	80
Brown rice, popcorn, oatmeal cookies	79
Sweetcorn, oat bran, buckwheat	78
Banana, sweet potato, Special K	77

Table 1.2 lists low Glycemic Index foods – these will help you avoid heart diseases, strokes, diabetes, obesity, intestinal cancer and low energy states.

TABLE 1.2 *Low Glycemic Index foods*

Low Glycemic Index foods	GI
Kiwi, Bran Buds	75
Canned kidney beans	74
Orange juice	74
Yam	73
Ice cream (low fat), Tortellini cheese	71
Black chocolate, carrots	70
Grapefruit juice, mixed grain bread	69
Green peas, oat bran bread	68
Grapes, pineapple juice	66
Yakult (fermented milk), lactose	64
Orange	63
Barley chapati, black gram	61
Chickpeas (canned), fresh peach, All Bran	60
Apple juice	59
Pinto beans	55
Apple	54
Fresh pear	53
Yoghurt (with no sugar added)	52
Milk 2%	48
Garbanzo beans	47

Low Glycemic Index foods	GI
Nutella spread	46
Yellow split peas (boiled)	45
Apricots (dried), butter beans	44
Soy milk, black beans	43
Green lentils, kidney beans	42
Sausages	40
Chapati (chickpea flour), Besan	39
Milk (full fat)	39
Spaghetti (protein enriched)	38
Lungkow bean thread	38
Grapefruit, red lentils, barley (pearled)	36
Brown beans (South African)	34
Fructose, cherries, dried peas	31
Rajman (red kidney beans)	27
Soybeans (canned), peanuts	21
Bengal gram dal (chana dal)	12
Nopal (prickly pear) cactus	10

Sugars in general

Listed below are some important and helpful facts and suggestions concerning all sugars:

- **Less fiber, less healthful.** Foods that are high in fiber (fruits; all vegetables except cooked carrots, beets and potatoes; all beans; salads) slow the absorption of sugar and, therefore, prevent insulin surge. So, to stay healthy and trim, avoid these low fiber "whites":
  - white rice
  - white flour (breads, pastries, cookies, biscuits)
  - white sugar
  - potatoes

  as *all* will be converted into saturated fats (TGs) and increase cholesterol, both of which clog the arteries.

- Some foods high in **fats** (e.g. whole milk) have a more healthful/lower GI (GI = 39) because fats slow the emptying of the stomach leading to the sugars being more slowly absorbed and thereby causing less of an insulin surge. In a word, the body's DNA recognizes whole milk as an ancient ally.

- If there is **too much sugar in the blood** the body protects the brain by converting the excess sugar to triglycerides (TGs).
- When you are **exercising regularly**, you increase the muscles' ability to extract the blood sugar from the bloodstream without the help of insulin.
- **Refined** (man-made) **sugar is strictly energy** (requiring exercise to prevent body fat deposition), devoid of vitamins and minerals, thereby sapping the body's reserves.
- **Sugar feeds yeast** (causing increased infections), blocks Vitamin C functions, and causes premature aging (by cross-linking reparative proteins).
- **Stop calling sugary foods "sweets"**. That causes mental confusion between your sweetheart and these "poisons". Call them "sugar bombs".
- **Beware hidden sugars**. The best rule of thumb for detecting fast hidden sugars is check the label for words ending in –ose, particularly those wrapped in bright red to get kids' attention: these include most commercial breakfast cereals, soft drinks (including sugary "fruit drinks"), baked goods, snacks, fast/junk foods (pizza, burgers, chips, crisps) and condiments. We are still familiar with the old adage "Just a spoonful of sugar helps the medicine go down," but we are consuming several cups per day. That leads to all sorts of health imbalances, low energy states and disease.

Fats: Tasty Villains or Lifesavers?

Fats have got an undeservedly bad name for themselves. As seen on the time line in Fig. 1.4, we have had an extremely productive relationship with fats since time immemorial (the same cannot be said for rapid sugars).

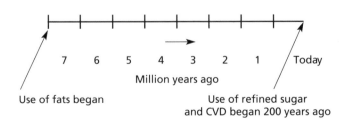

FIGURE 1.4 *Time line showing our relationship with fats and sugars*

So why the confusion? Just as sugar is a family of compounds (glucose, fructose, lactose), so too is fat. The scientific (and more precise) name for fats in the body is triglycerides: three (tri-) fatty acids attached to a glycerol backbone (glyceride).

Fats have got an undeservedly bad name for themselves

The most important aspect of the fatty acids is how many *double bonds* (i.e. unsaturation) exist between the carbon atoms. Saturated fats have no double bonds, while unsaturated fats have between one (mono-unsaturated) and six double bonds (the more double bonds, the better health-wise).

Saturated Fatty Acids

Saturated fatty acids have the following general properties:

- They do not react readily with other molecules: they are sluggish molecules (due to low molecular flexibility) that clog arteries when taken in excess.[17]
- They have a high melting point: solid at room temperature (blood becomes thicker and stickier).
- When incorporated into artery cell membranes, rigidity ensues and arteries stiffen.
- Saturated fatty acids are found in beef, lamb, pork, butter, certain cheeses, lard.
- These fats are used mostly as an energy source. When taken in excess, triglycerides in the blood increase and are stored as body fat.

Figure 1.5 shows stearic acid as an example of a saturated fatty acid (note the complete absence of double carbon bonds, so it is *completely saturated*). Therefore, it is solid at room temperature and, in excess, it will clog arteries.

Omega end[18]   Delta end

$$- C - C - C - C - C - C - C - C - C - C - C - C - C - C - C - C - C - C = O$$

$$|$$

$$OH$$

FIGURE 1.5 *A saturated acid molecule: note the absence of double bonds (=) between carbon atoms (C)*

Unsaturated Fatty Acids

Unsaturated fatty acids have the following general properties:

- They are flexible due to double bonds: they are highly reactive with other molecules.
- They have a low melting point: *always* liquid at room temperature (blood stays fluid and arteries stay supple).
- Mono-unsaturated fats (one double bond) are found in olives, olive oil, almonds, avocado, peanuts, cashews and filberts.
- Poly-unsaturated fats (more than one double bond).

Essential fatty acids

Essential fatty acids are *not* made by the body, therefore they must come from various foods. They include these two lifesavers:

- Linoleic acid (LA, with two double bonds): found in safflower, sunflower, sesame, flax, hemp, soybean, walnuts, pumpkin oils or 1–2 tablespoons of pure oil/day.
- Alpha linolenic acid (A-LNA, with three double bonds): found in flax, hemp, pumpkin seed, canola, soy oils, and walnuts or 1–2 teaspoons of pure oil/day.

Researchers now believe that both LA and A-LNA intersperse O_2 in the membranes with the following important implications:

- to act as a "microbial barrier" to invaders, such as viruses, bacteria and fungi;
- to delay lethargy, by clearing lactic acid after intense activity.

Super-Unsaturated Fats: Eicosapentaenoic Acid (EPA) and Docosahexanoic Acid (DHA)

These special oils are super-unsaturated and are found in cold-water fish such as sardines, mackerel, trout, herring and salmon. The oils are critical as they have been shown to incorporate themselves into the membrane of the mammalian heart muscle, thereby helping to stabilize erratic heart beats. Furthermore, these oils also lower blood pressure, triglycerides (by up to 65%), cholesterol (by a total of 25%), increase HDL and reduce platelet stickiness and inflammatory reactions.

Another potentially beneficial effect of these fish oils is that as they become incorporated into capillary cell membranes, they render the membranes more flexible. The result is that the red blood cells can flow more easily in tiny vessels.

These fats are used mostly in strategic metabolic functions, including the brain synapses, hormones, nerve conduction, arterial suppleness and reproductive organs. Figure 1.6 shows eicosapentaenoic acid as an example of a super-unsaturated fat (note the presence of five double bonds explaining *all* the beneficial aspects of these oils).

Omega[16] end   Delta end

$$- C - C - C = C - C - C = C - C - C = C - C - C = C - C - C = C - C - C - C - C = O$$
$$|$$
$$OH$$

FIGURE 1.6 *An unsaturated acid molecule: note the plenitude of double bonds (C = C)*

To conclude this section on fats, it is clear that for optimal health and longevity, you need to begin to shift your fat intake from the saturated (clogging fats) to the unsaturated fats, especially the mono-unsaturated and the super-unsaturated fats (cleaning fats).

The Cholesterol Family: Undeserved Calumny?

Total cholesterol = HDL cholesterol + LDL cholesterol + VLDL cholesterol

Just as sugar represents a family of compounds (glucose, fructose, lactose), so too does cholesterol. Hence, it makes absolutely no sense whatsoever just to discuss total cholesterol. Each member of the cholesterol family is a critical player in the fields of health and disease. We will look at each one in turn.

Each member of the cholesterol family is a critical player in the fields of health and disease

High Density Lipoprotein (HDL)

Some facts about HDL:

■ Desired blood value > 0.50 grams/liter (> 0.50 mgs/dl or > 1.3 mmol/liter).

- *Inversely* related to CAD (the higher the HDL, the lower the incidence of heart disease).
- HDL transports cholesterol away from the cells of the coronary arteries to the liver for processing and elimination (known as the "clean-up friend" of the arteries).

As to what makes the HDL go up, there's lots of good news here:

- Mediterranean diet: it's proven and correlates well with extended vitality and longevity in this region. Moreover, people who eat primarily a Mediterranean diet (rich in fruits, olive oil, fish, onions, garlic, red wine, beans) have been shown to have 70% less chance of a second heart attack compared to people on traditional northern European diets.[19]
- Eliminating refined sugars, as insulin suppresses HDL production.
- Giving up smoking, including passive or secondhand smoking.
- Essential fatty acids LNA + LA + EPA/DHA (fish).
- Shellfish (e.g. shrimp) actually raise the *good* cholesterol, HDL.[20] Shellfish contain two chemicals: chondroitin (blocks the enzyme that destroys cartilage) and glucosamine (stimulates cartilage growth) that offer some relief to arthritis sufferers.
- While up to three of any alcoholic drinks[21] (fermented, brewed, or distilled) is beneficial, red wine is ideal due to the blood-thinning properties of antioxidants (see Chapter 3).
- Physical activity: walking is ideal.

Triglycerides (TGs)

Some facts about TGs:[22]

- TGs are the fat we eat and store and, as such, represent a risk factor for heart disease.
- Desired blood value < 1.40 grams/liter (< 140 mgs/dl or < 1.6 mmol/liter).[23]
- *Directly* related to CAD (the higher the TGs, the higher the incidence of heart disease).
- Insulin converts refined sugar (and other foods with high Glycemic Indices) into stored TGs (stored body fat %).

- The TG:HDL ratio (in grams/liter) is one of the strongest predictors of heart disease, even stronger than the LDL:HDL ratio[24] (see Fig. 1.7). Recent studies found that elevated triglycerides increase the risk of heart attack even if the total cholesterol is normal.[25]
- Moreover, the Quebec Cardiovascular Study found that men with elevated TGs/LDL *plus* low HDL had 4.4 times the risk of a heart attack compared to those men without these risk factors.

TGs go up when there are high levels of inactivity or insulin. The best way to combat this is as follows:

- walking, walking, walking every day works best.
- low Glycemic Index foods and red wine, champagne, cognac or apple cider.

Important health note: the best single predictor for heart disease is the TG:HDL ratio in grams per liter, which should ideally be below 1. Up to 2 is acceptable and beyond 5 is the highest risk quintile.[26]

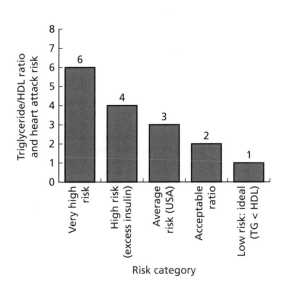

FIGURE 1.7 *TG:HDL ratio as indicator*

Low Density Lipoprotein (LDL)

Some facts about LDL:

- Desired blood value < 1.30 grams/liter (< 130 mgs/dl or < 0.5 mmol/liter).
- *Directly* related to CAD (the higher the LDL, the higher the incidence of heart disease).
- LDL transports cholesterol to the cells of the coronary arteries from the liver for arteriosclerotic plaque formation (it "clogs the arteries").

What makes the LDL go up (and what works best to lower it)?

- High intake of saturated fats, such as lamb, beef, pork, butter – prefer fish, poultry and game meats, such as venison.
- Body fat in excess of 20% for men and 23% for women – low sugar/ GI foods and walking.
- High GI foods – indirectly sends signal to the liver to make more LDL.

Vegetarianism: a personal choice

Neither abstinence from fish or flesh, nor going naked, nor shaving the head, nor wearing matted hair, nor dressing in rough garment, nor covering one with dirt, nor sacrificing to Agni, will cleanse a man who is not free from delusions. Anger, drunkenness, obstinacy, bigotry, deception, envy, self-praise, disparagement, superciliousness and evil intentions constitute uncleanness, not verily the eating of flesh.The self-indulgent man is a slave to his passions ... but to satisfy the necessities of life is not evil. To keep the body in good health is a duty, for otherwise we shall not be able to trim the lamp of wisdom and keep our minds strong and clear.

SAYINGS OF THE BUDDHA

In terms of prevention of disease, the research is compelling. Of all the research studies on the link between vegetable and fruit intake and cancers examined by the American Institute for Cancer Research, 78% demonstrated that vegetables and fruits are cancer preventative.

For the non-vegetarian, special care should be made to find a balance. There are far fewer nutrition issues with vegetarianism than with meat eating. According to the Worldwatch Institute, to produce 1 lb (500 grams) of steak costs the world 2 kilograms of grains, about 10,000 liters of water, 4 liters of gasoline and 15 kilograms of eroded topsoil. In order to make more grazing land for cattle, the tropical rain forest – a vital source of oxygen and a treasure chest of natural medicines for mankind – is destroyed at the rate of 4% per year. High temperatures and long cooking hours will "kill" the vitamins and enzymes in the food.

If you are a novice vegetarian, start easy and research the field thoroughly. Animal protein, though very costly from an ecological and health point of view, does indeed provide nutrients not immediately obvious to the new vegetarian – strive for balance.

The Dietary Pyramid Updated for The New Millennium

In contrast to certain governmental food pyramids (which at best represent a mixture of science and politics), the following food pyramid (shown in Fig. 1.8) incorporates strictly the scientific findings and their logical extrapolations, without a stitch of deference to the politics of the situation.[27]

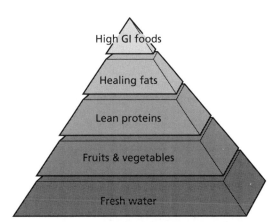

High GI foods
Beer, table sugar, potato, white rice, white bread, white flour

Healing fats
Oils: flax, hemp, soy, canola, saltflour, sunflower
Fatty fish: salmon, mackerel, herring
Olives, avocado, nuts, seeds

Lean proteins
Poultry, fish, yoghurt, soy, meats, cheeses

FIGURE 1.8 *Sensible food pyramid*

Foods with a high Glycemic Index (GI) are associated, especially when combined with low-fiber cereals, with diabetes[28] and heart disease,[29] via the mechanisms already discussed in this chapter (high insulin provoked by high GI foods leading to high TGs, low HDL and high overall TG/HDL ratio). At the McGannon Institute of Proactive Health (MIPH), we are involved in further research on the health effects of whole grains, fiber, sugar and fats of all kinds on the vitality, health and longevity of managers. Of special note in this pyramid is the importance of distinguishing between the cleaning fats (most oils) and clogging fats (most animal fats), as well as differentiating between healthful sugars (low GI) and harmful sugars (high GI).

Special research has been undertaken to include beneficial aspects of the Asian (Indian and Chinese) and Mediterranean diets, as the critical role of diets in the prevention of heart disease has contributed to the quality and length of life in these regions. Photocopy this pyramid (Fig. 1.8) and put it up on the fridge.

The French Diet: Integrating It All So Deliciously

Though the French diet has a relatively high fat content, the fats are all the beneficial ones: mono-unsaturated oils from the olive oil, antioxidants from the tomatoes, garlic, onions, wine and vegetables, and so-called cleaning fats (because they actually clean out the arteries: EPA/DHA) from the salmon, sardines, mackerels and herrings.

Table 1.3 gives you some suggested French menus but, in addition, we have supplied other menus from around the world for your pleasure and health (Tables 1.4–1.6). All these tables look at the following three categories that affect healthful nutrition:

- *Glycemic Index*: any GI greater than 75 will provoke insulin surges and should be avoided.
- *Fats present*: cleaning (if unsaturated) versus clogging (if saturated).
- How much compensation required: minutes of *metabolic walking* after the meal, on the basis of the GI and the fats present.

TABLE 1.3 *French menus*

Food on menu	Glycemic Index	Fats present	Post-meal walking required (minutes)	Comments
Marinated salmon mixed salad	Low ☺	Cleaning ☺	10	Perfect: use olive oil & lemon
Avocado stuffed with shrimp & scallop salad	Low ☺	Cleaning ☺	10	The cholesterol in shrimp is HDL!
Roasted lamb with beans	Beans = 42	Clogging ☹	15	Cook with garlic
Beef stew with carrots	Carrots = 70	Clogging ☹	15	With green salad for more fiber
Steak and French fries	Fries = 107	Clogging ☹	25	Dump the fries or add large green salad for more fiber
Pork chop with lentils	Lentils = 42	Clogging ☹	15	With garlic and parsley
Roasted rabbit with pasta	Pasta = 38	Cleaning ☺	15	Use olive oil
Grilled lamb kidneys with green beans	Low ☺	Clogging ☹	10	Use olive oil instead of sour cream
Chicken (without skin) sautéed with with green peas	Low ☺	Cleaning ☺	15	Cook chicken with cashew nuts
Steak tartar with mixed salad	Low ☺	Clogging ☹	10	Onions simmered in soy sauce
Broiled salmon with white rice	Rice = 128	Cleaning ☺	20	Savor the grilled salmon skin
Trout with almonds and steamed potatoes	Potatoes = 93	Cleaning ☺	20	Use olive oil instead of butter
Fried fish with fried vegetables	Low ☺	Clogging ☹	15	With salad and spinach for antioxidants
Tuna with tomatoes, onions & mushrooms	Low ☺	Cleaning ☺	10	Marinate tuna in olive oil, lemon, garlic
Mussels with wine & onions and seafood salad	Low ☺	Cleaning ☺	10	Serve with chilled Chardonnay

TABLE 1.4 *Chinese menus*

Food on menu	Glycemic Index	Fats present	Post-meal walking required (minutes)	Comments
Chinese soup with chicken & vegetables	Low ☺	Cleaning ☺	10	Chicken without skin
Shrimp with hot sauce & vegetables	Low ☺	Cleaning ☺	10	With cashew nuts
Chicken with peanuts & fried vegetables	Low ☺	Cleaning ☺	15	Stir-fry in sesame oil
Spicy fried rice with vegetables	Rice = 128	Cleaning ☺	20	With garlic and coriander
Lacquered duck with vegetables	Low ☺	Clogging ☹	15	Avoid skin of duck
Pork & fried rice	Rice = 128	Clogging ☹	25	With plenty of spinach for fiber
Roasted suckling pig with vegetables	Low ☺	Clogging ☹	15	Eat vegetables stir-fried and crunchy
Tom yam kung (spicy prawn soup & lemon grass)	Low ☺	Cleaning ☺	10	Serve with fresh coriander
Vegetarian spring roll	Low ☺	Cleaning ☺	15	Serve with chilled wine and spicy dressing
Chinese soup with pork & noodles	Noodles = 83	Clogging ☹	25	Walking and red wine can compensate

TABLE 1.5 *Indian menus*

Food on menu	Glycemic Index	Fats present	Post-meal walking required (minutes)	Comments
Kabab-E chaman (Spinach & lentils griddled fried)	Low ☺	Cleaning ☺	10	Serve with fresh onions and chickpea chapati
Aloo lajawab (Potatoes with mint & spices)	Potatoes = 93	Cleaning ☺	15	Serve with raw vegetables, like cucumbers, carrots and onions
Kandahari pulao (Rice with almonds & raisins)	Rice = 128	Cleaning ☺	15	Almonds high in Vitamin E and fiber
Dum-biryani (Steamed lamb & rice with spices)	Rice = 128	Clogging ☹	20	At least it is steamed! Serve with spinach
Rogan josh (Lamb cooked in a traditional gravy)	Low ☺	Clogging ☹	15	Serve with peanuts and fresh onions
Jhinga curry (Prawns cooked in an Indian curry)	Low ☺	Cleaning ☺	15	With almonds in olive oil
Tandoori bateyr (Farm-raised quails)	Low ☺	Cleaning ☺	10	With nuts and raisins
Seekh kabab gilafi (Lamb with tomatoes & onions)	Low ☺	Clogging ☹	15	Serve with spinach and cheese
Tandoori murgh (Half a chicken marinated in spices)	Low ☺	Cleaning ☺	10	Serve with a dry chilled white wine
Jhinga kesari (Saffron-flavored tandoori prawns)	Low ☺	Cleaning ☺	10	Serve with dal and palak

TABLE 1.6 *Indonesian/Malaysian menus*

Food on menu	Glycemic Index	Fats present	Post-meal walking required (minutes)	Comments
Udang serimpi with vegetables (Prawns in nut sauce)	Low ☺	Cleaning ☺	15	Lots of vegetables and a little rice
Sayor lodeh with steamed rice (Vegetables in coconut sauce)	Rice = 128	Clogging ☹	20	Coconut + rice = high saturation + high GI
Dalcha kambing with beans (Lamb dalcha)	Low ☺	Clogging ☹	15	With Bordeaux/ Burgundy wine
Udang sambal petai with beans (Prawns in bean sauce)	Low ☺	Cleaning ☺	15	Serve with vegetables
Daging masak merah with vegetables (Beef in red sauce)	Low ☺	Clogging ☺	15	With Bordeaux/ Burgundy wine
Sambal sotong with vegetables (Squid in spicy sauce)	Low ☺	Cleaning ☺	10	Serve with white wine
Sotong masak lemak with rice (Squid in coconut curry)	Rice = 128	Clogging ☹	15	Coconut + rice = high saturation + high GI
Ikan masak tempoyak (Fish in durian sauce)	Durian = high	Cleaning ☺	15	With spinach + walking!
Ayam masak merah with vegetables (Chicken in red sauce)	Low ☺	Cleaning ☺	10	Without skin
Kari ayam with rice (Chicken curry)	Rice = 128	Cleaning ☺	20	Coconut + rice = high saturation + high GI

TIPS FOR YOUR HEALTH ACTION PLAN

The best cocktail snack ... olives, nuts, almonds, cashews, cheese

The best cooking oil ... butter (more stable and less free-radical-producing than unsaturated oils), olive oil, palm oil

The best eating oil ... hemp, flax, olive, safflower

The best alcoholic drink ... red wine, white wine, champagne, cognac, armagnac, cider

The best non-alcoholic drink ... sparkling water, kiwi/carrot juice, fresh lime/lemon juice (without sugar), tomato juice

The worst alcoholic drink ... mixers

The best fat-burning exercise ... brisk walking after meal

The best animal protein ... cold-water fish (salmon, mackerel, herring, tuna)

The best vegetable protein ... soy, tofu, nuts, lentils, beans

The best way to increase TG/HDL ratio ... eat sugar (high Glycemic Index) and stay sedentary

The best snacks for children ... raw vegetables (celery, carrots) and fruits (apple) with peanut butter, nuts, dried fruits

The best way to extend life and maintain vitality ... walk, eat pure foods, and sleep well

The best way to gain 5 kilos ... go on a two-week holiday in Goa, drink beer, laugh all day and watch spectacular sunsets

The best way to lose 5 kilos ... exchange all that beer for two glasses of red wine daily for two months and walk daily

Frequently Asked Questions

Nutrition, Insulin and Health

Q What is the problem with **fast (junk) food**?

■ There are several important facts regarding Americans and junk food.[30] American rates of obesity have ballooned over the past 25 years (in 1960, 24% overfat; 1990, 35% overfat; by 2025, 65% estimated overfat). More and more junk food is being consumed:

$6 billion in 1970, $100 billion in 2000. Also consumed are high Glycemic Index (GI) foods:

- *French fries (chips)*: GI of 107 (one of the highest). In 1960, the average American ate almost 2 kilograms of frozen French fries per year. In 2000, the figure is almost 15 kilograms of French fries.

- *Sugar bombs*: Americans have abandoned water in favor of sugar drinks (the average can of cola contains the equivalent of ten tablespoons of refined sugar (GI = 137)). Consumption has increased since 1960 by more than 500%.

Remember: fast food = slow digestion = fast death. Besides the nutritive aspects which are, at best, dubious, fast (junk) foods are best perceived as "glue" for the digestive track, in that they are uniformly low-quality, low-fiber, highly refined foods that slow the transit time through the gut.

There is more to this plague. Everyone in society requires cultural guidelines. The loss of rituals can have a devastating effect on mental and physical health. In the moral sense, since we have largely abandoned the transmission of life's lessons from parent to child, the child has had to derive life's lessons from an infinitely more dangerous source: television (uninvited strangers in your home would be safer sources of influence). Instead of holding our elders in high esteem as vessels of wisdom, they are shipped off to "retirement institutions." Unfortunately for the family, they take their vast experience and wisdom with them. They don't call it "junk food" for nothing!

Q Can **medications** cause potential problems with cholesterol or insulin?

- *Diuretics* may elevate cholesterol and beta blockers can raise TGs and lower HDL. Both can worsen glucose intolerance.[31]

Q Is the **distribution of body fat** important?

- The Greeks understood this issue when they classified people into android distribution (apple-shaped) and gynoid distribution (pear-shaped). In 1983, understanding of the importance of the waist-to-hip ratio (WHR) was greatly improved.[32]

Important health note: an increase in WHR is closely correlated with increased intra-abdominal fat detected by CT scan.[33] In one study, for each 1% increase in this WHR over ideals, there was a 4% increase in mortality, due, in large part, to the mechanisms cited as follows:

Android (WHR > 0.95)	**Gynoid** (WHR < 0.85)
↑ Diabetes	No diabetes
↑ TGs, ↓ HDL	Normal TGs/ HDL
↑ BP	Normal BP
Result: ↑ CAD, shorter life	Result: ↓ CAD, longer life

Q Is there a **health risk with the body fat** by itself or with the associated syndromes?

■ If the excess body fat is *not* accompanied by high BP (>140/90), diabetes (blood sugar > 120 mg/dl), or high TGs (TGs > 1.40 g/l), there is *much* less risk of heart disease.[34] It still pays to be vigilant with excessive body fat, because isolated obesity remains quite rare.

Q How prevalent is **diabetes**?

■ Worldwide: 80 million (90% Type 2) (Europe 30 million, USA 17 million, India 22 million). The fate that awaits these cultures if no education is provided:

  – death due to coronary artery disease = 30%;

  – diabetes = first cause of blindness (< 50 years) in industrialized countries.

Q What is the most effective and quickest way to drop my blood level of **TGs**?

■ By avoiding high Glycemic Index foods (all refined sugars, white flour derivatives and white rice), and by walking 15 minutes after your heaviest meal, your TG level will drop by 50% within two to three months. By eating salmon and herring the effect you can achieve is even more dramatic.

Fats and Oils

Q Butter **or** margarine?

■ Trans fatty acids (used to increase the shelf life of cookies, crackers, biscuits, pastries and doughnuts, and also found in commercially fried foods) are derived from hydrogenated vegetable fats that go into margarine. They reduce cardio-protective HDL, increase LDL and are associated with heart disease and, possibly, cancer.

■ Butter tastes better, is more easily digested and contains calcium and Vitamin E. While butter causes increases in LDL, it causes increases in HDL as well. Check your numbers (TC, TGs, HDL, LDL) and stay as active as your grandparents were.

Q How often should I eat salmon to get enough super-unsaturated EPA/DHA?

■ The cardiovascular benefits of EPA/DHA last about ten days. Using fish that have these oils (EPA/DHA) once or, ideally, three times a week, will result in lower TGs, thinner blood, more supple arteries and, of course, less heart attacks. Hint: eat the skin; the oil is plentiful there!

The highest concentrations of EPA and DHA are found in all seafoods, particularly in cold-water fish. Atlantic mackerel lead the way (2,500 mgs/100 grams of raw fish), followed by Pacific salmon (1,500–2,500 mgs), albacore tuna (2,500 mgs), canned tuna (1,500 mgs), herring (1,600 mgs), rainbow trout (1,000 mgs), king crab (500 mgs), cod, snapper and shrimp (300 mgs), and, lastly, flounder, swordfish and lobster (200 mgs). The general rule of thumb is that the greater the amount of dark flesh on the fish, the greater the fat and omega-3 fatty acid content.

Q What are the best sources of the **essential fatty acids** (EFA)?

■ **Optimally balanced oils** have LA and LNA in balance: (in descending order) hemp oil, candlenut oil, chia oi, flax oil, wheat germ oil.

■ **Acceptably balanced oils** have LA but no LNA: (in descending order) evening primrose oil, safflower oil, sunflower oil, soybean oil, sesame oil.

Important health note: as the essential fatty acids are highly reactive, one must avoid contact with the elements that render the EFA ineffective: light, air and heat. Keep all oils containing EFAs in a cool dark place, such as the refrigerator.

Q Other uses of **olive oil**?

■ Researchers believe that olive oil may have the ability to help lower your risk of colon cancer. According to studies, it may be the high concentration of squalene, a constituent of olive oil, that lends olive oil its cancer-fighting powers.

Miscellaneous Topics

Q **Sandwiches**?

■ Make sure the bread is very high fiber (seed or nut bread). Too much commercial handling leads to increased risk of bacterial contamination.

Q What is the prevalence of **diabetes** in the USA?

■ Diabetes has risen 33%, from 4.9% to 6.5% of the population, with the greatest increase (70%) affecting 30–39 year olds. America's love-affair with sugars, inactivity and poor eating habits is causing this picture, which will, as in so many other aspects of modern life, be a negative model for other regions on the road to prosperity.

Q What are the **benefits of fish over meats**?

■ Fish, particularly caught in the wild, provides a source of lean protein, high super-unsaturated fats (which lower blood pressure), phosphorus, iron, copper and calcium (herring is exceptionally high in zinc). All fish provide anti-stress vitamins such as B vitamins. Fish help to prevent strokes by keeping the platelets from getting sticky and clumping. Take care not to destroy a great nutrition ally by overheating the fish.

Q I live five days a week in a **hotel** where the foods are inferior. What should I do?

■ Call the chef and explain your situation: he may empathize with you and be creative or you can change hotels. Second, buy bags of nuts (almonds, cashews, walnuts and hazelnuts) and dried fruits from a local health food shop. Munch on this mixture between meals to maintain stamina, blunt hunger and increase fiber to intestines. From your room, order a plate of fresh lemons and mineral water. Third, read Chapter 4: there is plenty there for every taste and speed.

Q Won't **walking after meals** put my heart at risk?

■ No, because the blood in the body will not be shunted from the heart for such a low-grade activity as brisk walking. As activity intensifies, the supply of the blood to the heart becomes more tenuous.

Q Lentils appear to be the ideal foodstuff. Why?

■ Lentils have been around for a long time (carbonated remains of lentils dating back 10,000 years, were discovered in Syria). They have the following benefits for health (see recipes in Chapter 3 also):

  – lean protein (used for antibodies, enzymes, muscles);

  – low fat;

  – zero cholesterol;

  – low Glycemic Index;

  – high fiber (helping to clear cholesterol and prevent colon cancer);

  – high in folate (more of this vitamin than any other unfortified food);

  – plenty of B vitamins: for proper brain functioning.

Q Is there a **body fat level** that is too low?

■ When women athletes get down to 5% or so, menstruation stops, which means they are no longer losing iron. Men at these levels report losing their libido.

Q Is there a relationship between being **overeating** and **cancer**?

■ In the Cardiovascular Health Study, involving nearly 6,000 people over the age of 65, those people with increased waist-to-hip ratios, body fat and elevated insulin levels are at least twice as likely to develop colon cancer than people without these findings.

SELF-ASSESSMENT QUIZ ▶▶▶▶

1 Body fat % should not exceed:

  (a) 10–13%
  (b) 15–20%
  (c) 21–23%

  Hint: Body compartments and density

2 Dieting (calorie deprivation) is clearly the best and most efficient way to control body fat:

  (a) True
  (b) False

  Hint: Metabolic rate

3 What is the best way to burn excess body fat?

   (a) Low-intensity exercise (walking)
   (b) High-intensity exercise (sprinting/squash)

   Hint: Oxygen availability

4 Losing excess body fat lowers blood cholesterol:

   (a) True
   (b) False

   Hint: The liver makes 80% of cholesterol from dietary and body fat

5 The low Glycemic Index foods can help control:

   (a) Body fat
   (b) High BP
   (c) High TC/LDL/TG
   (d) Blood sugar
   (e) Low HDL
   (f) Fatigue

   Hint: Insulin

6 It is better to eat fruits:

   (a) At the beginning of a meal
   (b) At the end of a meal
   (c) Between meals

   Hint: Fructose, water and fiber, and metabolic rate

7 Snacking promotes weight gain:

   (a) True
   (b) False

   Hint: Metabolic rate

8 It is easier to digest food when it is overcooked:

   (a) True
   (b) False

   Hint: Fast food = slow digestion = fast death

9 It is normal to feel tired after eating:

(a) True
(b) False

Hint: Food quality, walking and excess sugar

10 Muscle turns to fat when we stop using that muscle:

(a) True
(b) False

Hint: Metabolic rate

11 What are the caloric values of the following food groups (4, 7, or 9 calories/gram)?

(a) Proteins
(b) Carbohydrates
(c) Refined sugar
(d) Starch
(e) Fats and oils
(f) Alcohols

Hint: Insulin control instead of calorie counting

12 The best low Glycemic Index cocktail snacks include:

(a) Olives
(b) Nuts (peanuts, almonds, cashews …)
(c) Salty crackers
(d) Crisps (potato chips)

Hint: Insulin stores fat

13 The low GI alcoholic drinks include:

(a) Wine
(b) Beer
(c) Champagne
(d) Liqueurs

Hint: Grapes > grains

14 The best fats for health and longevity include:

(a) Essential fatty acids (flax, hemp, soy canola, safflower, sunflower)

(b) Super-unsaturated fatty acids (fatty fish)

(c) Mono-unsaturated fatty acids (olive, avocado, nuts, seeds)

Hint: Cleaning fats vs clogging fats

Answers

1 (b) for men	**10** (b)
(c) for women	**11** (a) = 4
2 (b)	(b) = 4
3 (a)	(c) = 4
4 (a)	(d) = 4
5 All	(e) = 9
6 (c)	(f) = 7
7 (b), depends on the GI of snack	**12** (a) & (b)
8 (b)	**13** (a) & (c)
9 (b)	**14** All

Notes

1 A new Japanese study, including more than 6,000 men, aged 35–60, found that men who reported walking between 11 and 20 minutes to work had a 12% reduction in hypertension and those who walked 21 minutes or more had a further drop in BP risk of 29% (*Annals of Internal Medicine*, 1999; 130: 21–6).

2 Recent findings suggest that high body fat in older age groups (>65 years) is associated with mobility-related disabilities (*American Journal of Clinical Nutrition*, 1998, Sep.; 68(3): 584–90).

3 Low-grade activity because any activity of higher intensity, such as jogging, would compromise the limited blood supply during digestion and result in digestive symptoms (bloating, bellyaches, and indigestion).

4 McArdle, W.D. et al., *Exercise Physiology. Energy, nutrition and human performance*, 1986.

5 More proof that walking is the best exercise: a recent study demonstrated that men aged 61–81 who walked more than 3 kilometers per day had a 50% decrease in cancer and overall death rate over men who walked less than a kilometer a day (Hakim, *New England Journal of Medicine*, 1998, Jan.).

6 *Circulation* (Journal of the American Heart Association), 2000, July.

7 Knopp et al., *Journal of the American Medical Association*, 1997; 278.

8 See Epilogue for a discussion of the 6Ws applied to the case study of the 100 most dire Mr Timebombs.

9 According to data from metabolic and epidemiologic studies of heart-disease risk and cholesterol, a decrease in saturated fat intake by 5% of energy would reduce heart disease rates by approximately 7%, and even less if the saturated fats are replaced by sugars with high Glycemic Index.

10 In fact, taking in 1000 mgs/day increases the blood cholesterol level by 5%.

11 Christensen, N.J., "Acute effects of insulin on cardiovascular function, noradrenaline uptake and release," *Diabetologia*, 1983; 25: 377–81.

12 Lever, A.F., "Slow pressor mechanisms in hypertension, a role for hypertrophy of resistance vessels?" *American Journal of Hypertension*, 1986; 4: 515–24.

13 Robertson, J.I.S., Fraser R., "Salt, volume and hypertension: causation or correlation?" *Kidney International*, 1987; 32: 590–602.

14 Landsberg, L., "Insulin sensitivity in the pathogenesis of hypertension," *J. Clin. Exp. Hypertens.*, 1996; 18 (3&4): 337–46.

15 In the Quebec Cardiovascular Study almost 70% of the people with heart disease had Syndrome X (elevated insulin as indicated by low HDL, high TGs/LDL) and for each 30% increase in insulin levels, there is a 70% increase risk of heart attacks over a five-year period.

16 The Glycemic Index (GI) is defined as the incremental area under the blood glucose response curve of a 50 gram carbohydrate portion of a test food expressed as a percent of the response to the same amount of carbohydrate from a standard food taken by the same subject. The GI tables here are based on testing with white bread. Either white bread or glucose can be used as the standard food. From Brand-Miller, Janette, "International tables of Glycemic Index," *American Journal of Clinical Nutrition*, 1995: 62 (supplement); 871S–893S.

17 The best way to see if you consume too much fat is to check your LDL cholesterol level, which should be less than 1.30 grams/liter.

18 The omega end is the point on the molecules from where we count the double bonds. Hence the expression "omega-3 fatty acid" signifies the presence of a double bond at position 3 from the omega end.

19 *Circulation* (Journal of the American Heart Association), 2000, Feb.

20 *American Journal of Clinical Nutrition*, 1998.

21 Recent analyses suggest that the increase of HDL accounts for about 50% of the protective effect of alcohol on coronary heart disease (see Gordon T. et al. "Alcohol and High Density Lipoprotein (HDL) cholesterol," *Circulation*, 1981; 64 (supplement II): II-63–III-67.

22 VLDL = TG/5.

23 Miller, *Journal of the American College of Cardiology*, 1998, May.

24 Gaziano J.M., *Circulation*, 1998, Oct. Gaziano and colleagues compared TGs and cholesterol levels in 340 cases of heart attack victims and an equal number of healthy persons. High TGs levels, combined with low HDL levels, were strongly associated with heart attack risk.

25 *Circulation*, 2000, June.

26 Gaziano J.M. et al., *Circulation*, 1998, Oct.

27 Note that the more we concentrate and distill foods, the less the body is equipped to deal with them. Examples include refined sugar, junk foods and distilled alcohol.

28 Salmeron J. et al., "Dietary fiber, glycemic load and risk of NIDDM in men," *Diabetes Care*, 1997; 20: 545–50.

29 Liu S. et al., "A prospective study of glycemic load and risk of myocardial infarction in women," *FASEB Journal*, 1998; 12: A260 (abstract).

30 Schlosser E., *Fast Food Nation,* Houghton Mifflin, 2001.

31 MacMahon, S.W. et al., "The effects of drug treatment for hypertension on morbidity/ mortality," *Prog. Cardiovasc. Dis.*, 1986; 29 (S1): 99–118.

32 Krotkiewski M. et al., "Impact of obesity on metabolism in men and women: importance of regional adipose tissue distribution," *Journal of Clin. Invest.* 1983; 72: 1150–62.

33 Ashwell M., *British Medical Journal*, 1985; 290: 1692–4.

34 Barrett-Connor, E.L., "Obesity, atherosclerosis and coronary heart disease," *Annals of Internal Medicine*, 1985; 103: 1010–19.

CHAPTER TWO

WATER

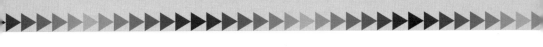

We started our existence in a maternal ocean and since our birth we have been in a constant state of dehydration, especially those of us who enjoy alcohol and coffee. Aging is a slow drying out process.

Using the advice contained in this chapter, Mr Timebomb could take care of the following health issues:

■ high uric acid
■ low stamina
■ rapid (inefficient) heart rate.

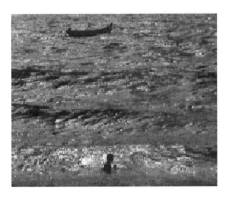

Why Is Water So Unique?

Some 200 to 300 million years ago, animals crawled up on to the land to have a look around. Our amphibious ancestors found life more interesting on dry land, adapted and stayed "topside," while the predecessors of other mammals (such as whales and dolphins) returned to the more stable environment of the seas.

Since that epoch, while living on the desiccated surface of our planet, we have become like "leaky" vessels, constantly losing vital fluids. We must now, therefore, carry our oceans with us.

The molecular structure and activity of water are unique. Life is not possible without this configuration of two hydrogen molecules and one oxygen molecule. This insignificant molecule has not merely changed the way we live life, it is the prerequisite for life itself.

> Up to 65% of your body's cellular mass is water;
> if you weigh 80 kilograms, that means you have about 50 kilograms
> of water molecules.

Some basic properties of water:

- Water is denser as a liquid than as a solid (ice floats). Imagine if water did not have this property.
- Water is a reasonable solvent.
- Boiling point of water = 100°C. Freezing point = 0°C. Density (specific gravity) = 1.0.
- Water ensures a stable environment.

Water and Health: Filters, Fruit and Fiber

Filters

Human beings interface with their environment by extracting what they need for survival and leaving the waste products behind. To extract the nutrients required for optimal health, the human body uses a series of filters:

- The kidneys filter the blood to maintain internal homeostasis by buffering acids and extracting water and minerals.

- The lungs filter the air, extracting oxygen and expiring carbon dioxide, to maintain the uninterrupted flow of oxygen to the brain.
- The digestive system extracts all essential nutrients (vitamins, minerals, calories, fats, sugar, protein) and calories.
- The mind filters experiences of life.

   As with any machine, to ensure their smooth working these filters must be cleaned up to remove any clogging residue. If the kidney does not filter the blood, waste products accumulate to a degree incompatible with life. If the lungs do not filter the air, we suffocate. If the gut does not filter our foods, we starve. If the mind does not filter experiences, we risk dying stupid.

The digestive system

The large intestine (colon), from 1–2 metres in length, is not involved in the digestion of nutritive chyme (see Fig. 2.1). It is in charge, rather, of

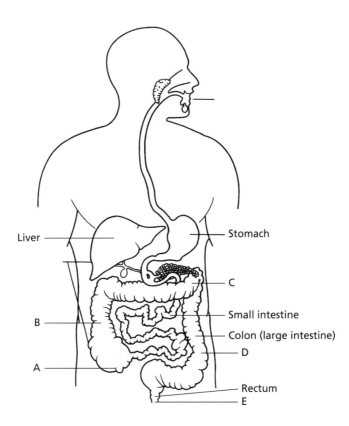

FIGURE 2.1 *The human digestive tract*

transforming the liquid chyme into solid faeces by absorbing the water and minerals. If water intake is too low, the colon will wring the chyme of water until the intestinal contents are hard and dry. This leads to constipation, a most undesirable condition in which waste products are retained until sufficient water is supplied.

Prolonged retention of faecal material and the attempts at forceful elimination thereof, could lead to a wide variety of intestinal ailments such as appendicitis (point A), spasm and painful distension and gas (point B), polyps (point C), diverticulosis (painful herniated outpockets through the muscular wall of the large intestine, point D), diverticulitis, colitis, hemorrhoids (point E) and, quite possibly, colon cancer. All this misery could be side-stepped by simply ensuring adequate water intake on a *regular* basis.

Fruit

In the task of optimizing health, **fruits** are vitally helpful for three reasons. They have, in abundance:

- *fiber* (roughage): naturally packaged vitamins;
- *fructose* (low Glycemic Index of 32);
- *water* (most fruits are 85–95% water).

You can avoid digestive problems (appendicitis, colitis, pre-cancerous polyps, colon cancer, diverticulosis, hemorrhoids and intestinal spasm) by consuming fresh fruit at will. If you are already plagued by unpleasant digestive problems (or, in fact, any health problem), it would be a good idea to do a fruit fast, thus cleaning the digestive filter. A fruit fast is a big clean out, a veritable digestive reset button to get back the health of your digestive track. It is ideally undertaken on a free day over the weekend:

You can avoid digestive problems by consuming fresh fruit

- Start with a glass of lemon water before and after your daily 4-minute workout. Then, settle down with a book, board games or mind-centering activity. Nibble on a whole-almond raisin-mixed snack throughout the morning, accompanied only by fresh fruits and lemon water.
- For lunch, add something salty like a simple soup or a green salad. Drink water freely, but no commercial fruit juice. Add a little Vitamin C (2 grams) to help the cleansing process along.

■ Expect a fulll evacuation of the intestines by early evening, accompanied by a feeling of energy and lucidity as the brain benefits from this very natural detoxification.

■ The following day, resume gradually the usual eating habits, starting with more coarse foods and moving slowly toward the more refined as per your new tastes. Using this physiologic "reset" button, you will easily be able to identify the foods that cause problems such as headaches, constipation, low energy and listlessness.

Fiber

Fiber, which acts as a "bottle brush" as it helps to move along the waste products of the intestines, has been associated with less constipation, reduced diverticular disease, and a decreased risk of colon (large intestine) cancer and heart disease. A six-year study of almost 44,000 male health professionals from 40 to 75 years of age showed that those who consumed the most fiber had 35% fewer heart attacks over the low-fiber controls. Moreover, in a large prospective study, breast cancer incidence was about 25% higher among women with a low intake of vegetables.

Fiber found especially in apples, pears, carrots, almonds, beans, oats, grains, cabbage, peas, tomatoes and kelp, can bind and eliminate cholesterol. In a recent study, people who consumed a high fiber diet were found to be less likely to develop increased insulin, high central body fat and diabetes.

Tables 2.1 and 2.2 provide a breakdown of the fiber/ vitamin loads present in a variety of fruits, nuts and seeds.

TABLE 2.1 *Fruits and their fiber/vitamin load*

Fruits	Quantity	Fiber (grams)	Glycemic Index	Vitamin E (international units)	Vitamin C (mgs)	Vitamin A (international units)
Apple	1	1.06	54	1.0	7.8	74
Apricot	3	0.64	82 (dried = 44)	–	10.6	2769
Avocado	1	4.24	–	–	15.9	1230
Banana	1	0.57	77	0.6	10.3	92
Cantaloupe	½ medium	0.97	93	3.0	112.0	8608
Currants, black	1 cup	2.69	–	–	202.0	258
Cherries	1 cup	0.58	32	–	6.1	310
Dates	10	1.83	146	–	0	42
Figs	1	0.77	–	–	1.3	91

Fruits	Quantity	Fiber (grams)	Glycemic Index	Vitamin E (international units)	Vitamin C (mgs)	Vitamin A (international units)
Grapefruit	1	0.24	36	0.26	41.3	149
Grapes	1 cup	0.72	66	–	17.3	117
Guava	1	5.04	–	–	165.0	713
Honeydew	1/10	0.77	–	–	32.0	52
Kiwi fruit	1	0.84	75	–	74.5	133
Kumquat	1	0.7	–	–	7.1	57
Lychee	1	0.2	–	–	6.9	–
Mango	1	1.73	80	3.0	57.3	8060
Melon, casaba	1/10	0.97	–	0.28	112.0	8608
Nectarine	1	0.54	–	–	7.3	1001
Orange	1	0.56	63	0.43	69.7	269
Papaya	1	2.35	–	–	187.0	6122
Passion fruit	1	1.97	–	–	5.4	126
Peach	1	0.56	60	–	5.7	465
Pear	1	2.32	53	–	6.6	33
Persimmon	1	2.49	–	–	12.6	3640
Pineapple	1 cup	0.84	94	–	23.9	35
Plantain	1	0.74	–	–	27.2	1668
Plum	1	0.4	55	–	6.3	213
Prune	10	1.72	–	–	9.0	2.8
Raisins	1 cup	1.11	91	–	9.0	
Raspberries	1 cup	3.69	–	–	30.8	160
Rhubarb	1 cup	0.85	–	–	9.8	160
Strawberries	1 cup	0.79	–	–	84.5	41
Watermelon	1 cup	0.48	103	–	15.4	585

Source: United States Department of Agriculture

TABLE 2.2 *Nuts and seeds and their fiber/vitamin/fat load*

nuts/ seeds	Quantity	Fiber (grams)	Vitamin E (IU)	Selenium (micro- grams)	Saturated fat (grams)	Unsaturated fat (grams)	Cholesterol (grams)
Almonds	1 cup	3.84	21.3	2.8	6.2	67.0	0
Brazil nuts	1 cup	4.2	9.1	144.0	18.7	69.3	0
Cashews	1 cup	1.96	–	–	10.9	49.3	0
Chestnuts	1 cup	0.8	0.8	–	0.44	2.04	0
Coconut	1 cup	2.7	0.8	–	24.3	2.0	0
Hickory nuts	15 small	0.3	28.0	2.7	0.9	8.8	0
Macadamia	1 cup	7.08	–	–	14.8	80.0	0
Peanuts	1 cup	3.89	9.36	–	15.4	50.5	0
Peanut butter	1 tablespoon	0.33	–	–	1.5	6.1	0

nuts/ seeds	Quantity	Fiber (grams)	Vitamin E (IU)	Selenium (micro-grams)	Saturated fat (grams)	Unsaturated fat (grams)	Cholesterol (grams)
Pecans	1 cup	2.3	1.5	3.24	5.4	63.8	0
Pine nuts	1 cup	0.31	–	–	1.7	11.7	0
Pistachios	1 cup	2.4	–	2.8	6.2	67.0	0
Pumpkin	1 cup	2.66	–	–	11.8	51.0	0
Sesame	1 cup	3.6	–	–	11.2	64.0	0
Sunflower	1 cup	5.5	–	–	8.2	59.6	0
Tahini	1 tablespoon	0.75	–	–	1.13	6.57	0
Walnuts	1 cup	2.1	1.5	–	4.5	49.5	0

Source: United States Department of Agriculture

Understanding foods

Exercise: modern fast foods may actually taste good during consumption but they may cost dearly in health terms. Don't make your arteries pay for the caprices of your palate. Match each food with its ingredients:

Modern fast foods may actually taste good during consumption but they may cost dearly in health terms

Food

1 Potato chips (crisps)
2 Diet soda drink (cherry)
3 "Natural" candy bar
4 Instant pancake mix
5 Dog food
6 Lite Italian salad dressing
7 Breakfast cereal

8 Instant soup
9 Colored candies for kids
10 "Natural" cookies ("less than 40% fat")
11 Throat lozenges
12 Instant tea drink
13 Isotonic drink

Ingredients

(a) Bleached flour (wheat flour, niacin, reduced iron, thiamine mononitrite, riboflavin), sugar, soy flour, leavening, vegetable shortening (partially hydrogenated soybean and cottonseed oils), dextrose, eggs, buttermilk, salt, soy lecithin (an emulsifier) and non-fat milk.

(b) Maltodextrin, malic acid, instant tea, aspartame (phenylalanine), natural lemon flavor.

(c) Sugar, butter, whole milk powder, cocoa mass, whey powder, lecithin (emulsifier), flavoring, may contain nut traces.

(d) Beef, mutton, poultry, bone, gels, food coloring, vitamins and minerals.

(e) Potatoes, palm oil, spices, salt, glutamic acid, citric acid.

(f) Carbonated water, sucrose, glucose, citric acid, sodium chloride, potassium phosphate, sodium benzoate, E211, Vitamin C, calcium phosphate.

(g) Sugar, corn syrup, dextrose, glycine, gelatin, artificial flavor, vegetable gums, colors including red 3, red 40 lake, blue 2 lake.

(h) Water, distilled vinegar, salt, sugar, less than 2% garlic, natural flavors, soybean oil, xanthan gum, sodium benzoate, potassium sorbate, calcium-disodium EDTA (preserves freshness), yellow 5, red 40.

(i) Wheat flour, palm and sesame oils, freeze-dried mushrooms, dehydrated sweetcorn, leeks, carrots, seaweed, sugar, monosodium glutamate (MSG).

(j) Corn, oat and wheat flours, vegetable oils (soy, cottonseed, sunflower), salt, sugar, natural colors (annattol, carmine).

(k) Enriched wheat flour, raisins, rolled oats, fructose, polydextrose, soybean oil, water, apple and pineapple juices, powered cellulose, corn syrup, dough conditioner (lecithin), less than 2% apples, corn starch, leavening agents, ammonium bicarbonate, bicarbonate of soda, sodium aluminium phosphates, natural and artificial flavors, spices, pectin, citric acid.

(l) Dextrose maltose, dextran corn syrup, malic acid, less than 2% artificial and natural flavors, calcium stearate, color additives, wax, blue 1, blue 1 lake, red 40 lake, yellow 5 lake, yellow 6 lake, yellow 6.

(m) Carbonated water, sugar, citric acid, sodium benzoate E211, caramel E150, colour (E122).

Answers:

1 (e)	**6** (h)	**10** (k)
2 (m)	**7** (j)	**11** (g)
3 (c)	**8** (i)	**12** (b)
4 (a)	**9** (l)	**13** (f)
5 (d)		

Caffeine

Caffeine is one of our civilization's stimulants of choice, but it deserves a better analysis as it tends to provoke marked disturbances in our internal homeostasis, particularly when combined with nicotine and alcohol.

Caffeine has the following physiologic effects:

- Long half-life[1] ($T_{\frac{1}{2}}$) of 5 hours, therefore tends to disturb sleep patterns.
- Excites the heart: increases blood pressure, heart/breathing rates.
- Increases the levels of the stress hormone adrenaline.
- Increases the levels of the stress hormone cortisol.[2]
- Diureses vital fluids: stimulates vitamin and mineral loss (B vitamins, iron, calcium,[3] zinc, magnesium) and water loss.
- Contributes to heartburn (reflux esophagitis), as caffeine allows the acidic stomach contents to escape.
- Causes increased acid secretion in stomach, leading to gastritis and ulcers.
- Possibly responsible for PMS symptoms (tension, irritability, anxiety, breast tenderness, insomnia).
- In *excess* (300–1000 mg), caffeine causes irritability, sleeplessness, anxiety, rebound depression, increased acid secretions and ulcers, irregular heart beats, dehydration and mineral deficiencies.

Table 2.3 shows the caffeine content of various foods and drugs.

TABLE 2.3 *Caffeine content of various foods and drugs*

Drink/Drug[4]	Range (mg)	Mean (mg)
Roasted/ground coffee (percolated)	64–124	83
Instant coffee	40–180	59
Decaffeinated coffee	2–5	3
Tea	8–91	27
Cocoa (African)	–	6
Cocoa (South American)	–	42
Cola drinks	12–19	15
Milk chocolate	–	40
Migril (one tablet)	–	100
Cafergot (one tablet)	–	100
Antoin (max. recommended dose)	–	120
Doloxene (max. recommended dose)	-	120
Cafadol (one tablet/capsule)	-	30
Hypon, Capol Extra (one tablet/capsule)	–	10

Caffeine dependence

Are you hooked on the most widely used psychoactive drug in the world? Be aware of *caffeine withdrawal syndrome* (headaches, irritability, insomnia and depression). In addition to the physical symptoms of withdrawal, researchers have added three other criteria for *substance dependence* under the DSM-IV:[5] persistent desire, dose tolerance and unsuccessful attempt to control use.

Are you hooked on the most widely used psychoactive drug in the world?

In order to free yourself of caffeine dependence, start by imagining your life without caffeine. Then taper off caffeine slowly, over, say, two weeks. After a week off caffeine, you will be your old refreshed self again, free of yet another false stimulant. Otherwise, caffeine should be kept "off limits" to heart and blood pressure patients, pregnant and breastfeeding women.

Why Tea is so Healthful

Tea (both green and black) not only has less energy-sapping caffeine, it is also a rich source of antioxidants called flavonoids. There is a growing body of evidence that confirms that these flavonoids play an important role in protecting us from heart disease and cancer.

Epidemiological studies suggest that tea consumption is associated with decreased cardiovascular disease risk, but the complete mechanisms of action remain incompletely elucidated. Clearly, the antioxidants in tea (flavonoids) have been shown to reverse artery dysfunction. Here's what is clear so far about this marvelous beverage:

1 Acute and chronic tea consumption *improves coronary arterial dilation* in patients with coronary artery disease.[6]

2 A single dose of tea with or without milk *increases plasma antioxidant activity* in humans.[7] Consumption of a single dose of black and green tea induces a significant rise in plasma antioxidant activity *in vivo*. The addition of milk to tea does not abolish this increase. Whether the observed increases in plasma antioxidant activity after a single dose of tea prevent *in vivo* oxidative damage remains to be established.

3 *Green tea* has many healthful ingredients, key among which is epigallocatechin gallate (EGCG), one of the most powerful members of the polyphenol antioxidant family of "catechins." This antioxidant, EGCG, neutralizes free radicals, blocks cell mutations and prevents tumor growth factors, particularly in rectal and intestinal cancer.

4 *Weight control*: a recent study from researchers in Geneva, Switzerland suggests that green tea both increases the metabolic rate and speeds up the burning of fat. The rate of thermogenesis (calorie burning) increased by nearly 5% in the groups of subjects drinking green tea extract.

TIPS FOR YOUR HEALTH ACTION PLAN

The best fiber snack ... almonds

The best drink ... water between meals

The best sleep inducers ... whole milk (warmed) with honey

The best time to drink water ... between meals (with fruits and nuts) and just before eating

The best water temperature ... room temperature (with a lime twist)

The best way to feel tired ... take three more cups of coffee per day and avoid physical activity

Frequently Asked Questions

Fiber and the Gut

Q How can I avoid **constipation**?

■ Do a fruit fast to achieve the *big clean out*. Then, maintain daily regularity with lemon water and an increased intake of fruit and nuts (especially well-chewed almonds).

Q What are the important components of **food labels**?

■ Generally, the nutritional information currently presented to the consumer is incomplete and inadequate for making intelligent decisions about health.

■ **Fiber**: very useful (the more the better).

■ **Glycemic Index**: critical, especially on products destined for children.

■ **Sugar**: listings of all sugars should be replaced by Glycemic Indices of all components of foods (the lower the better), to sidestep the confusing listings seen today: starch, sugar, carbohydrates.

- **Fats**: should include not just totals and % saturated but also the presence of super-unsaturated oils, such as EPA, DHA, and the essential fats, LNA and LA.
- **Protein**: useless.
- **Sodium**: useful for people with high blood pressure.
- **Antioxidants**: should definitely be listed.

Water and Caffeine

Q **Water** with meals: fizzy or flat?

- Do not drink serious amount of water with meals: sip only. It is better to sip wine with meals than water. Water, fizzy or flat (according to your taste), with a lemon added, should be drunk freely one hour after meals (allowing time for the stomach to empty), right up to the beginning of meals (as it empties *immediately* from the stomach).

Q Does **caffeine/alcohol** count as a water source?

- Not at all. *Au contraire*, they are diuretic (they make you urinate). Compensate with water and natural fruit juices.

Q Green tea vs black tea: **antioxidants**?

- Studies show that oolong and green teas may keep your teeth healthy by reducing the amount of plaque-causing bacteria in your mouth. The polyphenols in these teas appear to inhibit the formation of cavity-promoting bacteria.

Q Are **cola** drinks safe?

- Once a month poses no health threat. Soft drinks tend to contain phosphates, which accelerate calcium (bone) loss. They also contain caffeine, which gets everyone unnecessarily excited for no reason, including children. Drink carrot or kiwi juice.

Q Dried fruits? Fruit juice?

- Dried fruits should be rehydrated with several glassses of lemon water. Only natural juices (prepared by you in the morning in your juicer) are acceptable.

Q Uric acid and gout: what can be done?

■ If your uric acid is elevated, there is an 80% chance that you will be an under-excreter (who will respond nicely to liberalizing your water intake, as discussed) and a 20% chance that you are an overproducer (who will still benefit from water, but will need to look at nutrition as well, and possibly medication).

SELF-ASSESSMENT QUIZ

1 A decline in performance (physical and psychological) takes place when as little as _____ % of our total body water is lost:

(a) 5%
(b) 10 %
(c) 30%

Hint: The body is 65% water

2 Drinking water during your meal aids the digestion of food:

(a) True
(b) False

Hint: Dilution of gastric juices

3 Colas and beers replace water loss:

(a) True
(b) False

Hint: Caffeine and alcohol are diuretics

4 Fruit juices are optimal to drink all day long:

(a) True
(b) False

Hint: Water is best!

5 What is the half-life ($T_{\frac{1}{2}}$) of caffeine?

(a) 2 hours
(b) 5 hours
(c) 12 hours

Hint: Metabolic rate

6 It is better to eat fruits:

(a) At the beginning of a meal
(b) At the end of a meal
(c) Between meals

Hint: Fructose, water, fiber and metabolic rate

7 Drinking plenty of water (2–3 liters/day) can help avoid the following:

(a) Appendicitis
(b) Colitis
(c) Polyps
(d) Colon cancer
(e) Hemorrhoids
(f) Constipation
(g) Low energy states
(h) Flatulence

Hint: Fructose, water, fiber and metabolic rate

8 Eating plenty of fruits and vegetables can help replace water loss:

(a) True
(b) False

Hint: Fructose, water, fiber and metabolic rate

9 Which problems are caused by low fiber intake?

(a) Appendicitis
(b) Colitis
(c) Polyps
(d) Colon cancer
(e) Hemorrhoids
(f) Constipation
(g) Low energy states
(h) Flatulence
(i) Heart attack

Hint: Clean out the filter

10 Which waters are best?

(a) Mineral
(b) Sparkling
(c) Distilled

Hint: The body is 65% water

11 If you drank your last expresso (about 300 mg) at 3 pm, what would the blood concentrations of caffeine be at these hours?

(a) 8 pm _____ mg
(b) 1 am _____ mg
(c) 6 am _____ mg

Hint: Caffeine's long $T_{\frac{1}{2}}$ means that you may be on the drug permanently

12 The best way to know if you are dehydrated is:

(a) Check urine
(b) Thirst
(c) Skin tone
(d) Spittle color

13 Constipation increases the following health risks for:

(a) Intestinal cancer
(b) Heart disease
(c) Appendicitis

Answers

1 (a)	**6** (c)	**11** (a) =150
2 (b)	**7** All	(b) =75
3 (b)	**8** (a)	(c) =37.5
4 (b)	**9** All	**12** (a) & (d)
5 (b)	**10** All	**13** All

Notes

1 The half-life ($T_{\frac{1}{2}}$) is a clearance constant for each drug. It is defined as the time necessary to clear half the concentration of a particular drug. The long ($T_{\frac{1}{2}}$) means that the drug and its effects lingers around the clock. For example, if nicotine has a $T_{\frac{1}{2}}$ of 2 hours, the body will clear half of the nicotine in a cigarette smoked at 10 pm by midnight and half again (that is, a quarter of the original concentration) by 2 am.

2 Cortisol causes the heart to pump harder while constricting the blood vessels. See Shepard J.D.et al., *American Journal of Hypertension*, 2000, May. .

3 Osteoporosis is now becoming an adolescent problem, as kids are consuming sugary caffeine-containing drinks, such as colas. The sugar/caffeine combination causes marked calcium losses (from the bones) in the urine, from 16 mgs/hour to 30 mgs/hour. See Massey I.K., "Acute effects of dietary caffeine and sucrose in mineral excretion in healthy adolescents," *Nutr. Res.* 1988; 8(9).

4 Note: one cup = 150 ml and one mug = 200–230 ml. Source: British National Formulary, London; BMA and Royal Pharmaceutical Society, 1992.

5 *The American Psychiatric Association's Diagnostic and Statistical Manual of Mental Disorders*, 4th Edition.

6 Stephen J. Duffy, Boston University School of Medicine, Boston, MA; Balz Frei, Linus Pauling Institute, Corvalis, OR; Monika Holbrook, Peter Swerdloff, Elizabeth S. Biegelsen, Noyan Gokce, Ross M. Germani, Judson D. Russell, John F. Keaney Jr, Joseph A. Vita, Boston University School of Medicine, Boston, MA.

7 Leelan R., Roodenberg A.J.C., Tijburg L.B.M. & Wiseman S.A., *European Journal of Clinical Nutrition*, 2000; 54: 87–92.

CHAPTER THREE

WINE

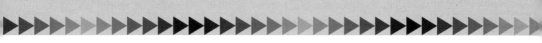

Wine, often referred to as the "drink of the gods," is extremely beneficial to your health and sanity.

The information in this chapter will enhance your health, vitality and longevity by resolving the following health issues:

- low HDL ("good") cholesterol
- thickened blood
- low stamina and energy
- LDL ("bad") cholesterol
- poor sleeping habits.

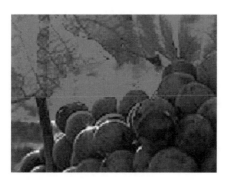

Early Uses of Alcohol[1]

Since *Homo sapiens* stood erect and developed the consciousness of himself as an isolated being, he has reserved the right to find ways to promote the kind of commonality that originally held together primitive tribal communities. In his search for this transcendence, he has discovered all sorts of substances (and ways to use these substances) to shift his awareness away from his aloneness. In fact, some ethnopharmocology anthroplogy researchers make very convincing arguments that the entire history of humankind throughout the ages has really been one of (clumsily at first, then with increasing efficiency and refinement) finding "cultural allies" or products that help to capture that eternal moment of commonality experienced by all of our ancestors while discussing, laughing and dancing around the campfire and intermittently gazing up at the stars.[2]

The earliest civilizations in Mesopotamia, China and Egypt stumbled eagerly upon fermented honey (mead), grains, sap and fruits, probably after watching the effect of these on birds, squirrels, bears and elephants.

Alcohol: Protector or Poison?

Humankind has been in a gyrating tryst with alcohol since 6000 BC. Only recently have we begun to really understand that something we enjoy as part of a ritual of celebration also has wonderfully beneficial effects on health and longevity. The issue of alcohol's impact on health and culture has been hotly debated in scientific research forums around the world, as neither scientist nor layperson can ignore the central paradox inherent in alcohol use. That is, while alcohol can produce a natural euphoria and promote health, it also has the dubious status as the substance that has had the most profoundly detrimental effects on humankind throughout history.

Keep an Eye on the Dark Side of Booze ...

Listed below are some of the detrimental effects of alcohol:

■ Alcohol is metabolized at a rate of roughly one unit or drink (half-pint of beer, a glass of wine or a shot of spirits) per hour, so after six drinks at 10 pm, the blood alcohol level and stuporous effects of the alcohol would be approaching nil by 4 am. As this happens, we experience a rebound hyperexcitation, accompanied by increased adrenaline levels in the blood, insomnia, higher blood pressure, rapid heart rate, sweating, headaches and nightmares.

- Alcohol is responsible, at least in part, for such scourges as slavery, domestic violence, accidents, poor sexual performance, low self-confidence, depression and suicides. It would be irresponsible to claim otherwise.
- Alcohol causes marked water and mineral losses.
- Alcohol can worsen borderline blood pressure problems.
- Alcohol is calorifically dense: 7.2 calories/gram.
- When alcohol is consumed on an empty stomach, 25% passes directly through the unprotected stomach lining.
- Alcohol is a brain depressant, which when used in excess to control stress can destabilize positive attitudes and relationships.
- Alchol can increase triglycerides.

. . . And Then Enjoy It

The bottom line is that when consumed in a relaxed way the verdict has been back for years: moderate consumption of alcohol can be a powerful preventative factor against heart disease.

Moderate consumption of alcohol can be a powerful preventative factor against heart disease

Why Wine is Unique

The so-called French Paradox

Wine comes in at the lips, love comes in at the eye,
So I raise my glass and look at thee and I sigh

The consumption of the juice of the fermented grape probably happened by chance some 8,000 years ago in Mesopotamia (present-day Iraq) and moved eastward at a rate commensurate with its ease of production and improving taste. Wine-growing technology arrived about 4,000 years ago in Greece, where it was exported to southern Italy by 1000 BC, hitting the Roman Empire (which had effective ways of storing wine in wooden barrels and glass bottles) just in time for distribution to the full extent of the empire: to Spain, Portugal, France and even Britain.

After the fall of the Roman Empire, fearing that the secret of wine would be lost during the Dark Ages in Europe, the Church (as a vast land owner) became intensely involved in wine cultivation, both as a product and as a way to know God (at least for the priests who imbibed during the Mass and the altar boys who did so afterwards). In fact, wine's sweep throughout Europe was greatly accelerated by the Christian monasteries that perceived a vested interest in cultivating wine. It was that same precious nectar that might some day be converted into the blood of Christ during the Mass, in the same way that Christ himself had transformed the water into wine at a Canaan wedding many centuries earlier.

Centuries later, in a moment in 1926 of particular lucidity, the Catholic Church in the USA announced its opposition to compulsory Prohibition, saying that Prohibition was contrary to the Bible and that wine had benefits "ranging from the supreme honor paid wine with bread, as the matter of the holy Eucharist, to its general work of moistening and enlivening the rough fare of laborers."

The folklore of wine has continued to the present day, fueled not only by the improved taste but also by reports that wine, particularly red wines, have mystical health powers. It is most particularly in France where we can see the confounding magic at work in the form of the French paradox.[3] Do the vaulted claims about wine's life-giving properties and beneficial effects on health and longevity have any basis at all in scientific fact? The answer is simple: yes.

Even with the proviso that alcohol (wine is roughly 14% alcohol) in excess leads to disease and death, the medical research is replete with studies that enthusiastically support the link between moderate (and regular) consumption of wine and the prevention of various diseases, most notably:

1 *Coronary artery disease* (CAD): scores of well-designed studies have demonstrated time and time again the protective effect of moderate red wine consumption against heart attacks, particularly in countries like France, where there is a high consumption of fat. In the UK, for example, recent studies have demonstrated that moderate red wine drinking could reduce the incidence of CAD by half! What is the mechanism of this natural magic? Wine decreases stress, makes platelets less sticky (although the effect is short-lived – 24 to 48 hours – so regular wine is better), increases HDL and makes the body more insulin sensitive[4] (hence, lower TGs and higher HDL).

2 *Strokes*: strokes account for a significant health burden worldwide. While two to three glasses per day of red wine reduces the risk of stroke, more than five to six glasses per day would actually increase the risk of cerebral hemorrhage due to the combined effects of increased blood pressure and less sticky blood.

3 *Diabetes mellitus* (DM): this disease afflicts more than 125 million people worldwide and can be easily treated with diet and low-grade exercise. Grapes have a much lower Glycemic Index (66) than the sugar in beer (maltose = 150) and, therefore, will not cause insulin surging that could lead to central obesity and, in turn, diabetes.

4 *Osteoporosis*: studies have shown that grape skins contain a natural estrogen-like chemical, called *resveratrol*, that not only keeps the platelets from forming a clot and reduces inflammation, but may act to make bones more massive and less prone to fractures. Moreover, as estrogen positively affects the HDL cholesterol and keeps artery linings smooth, this may help to explain yet another protective aspect of red wines.

5 *Cancers*: the oxidative process that plays such a critical role in cancer development is blocked by the antioxidants in red wine.

Which Reds are Best?

The best reds are those that have had the chance to soak in the skin of the grape. The powerful chemicals known as antioxidants reside in the skin, doing their job for the grape of protecting it from its own natural enemies: UV rays and fungi. There is an abundance (up to 100) of antioxidants in red wine (a far more plentiful source than white wine, in which the skin is discarded during the fermentation process), though the levels will vary with the grape and the year. Several rules of thumb hold for the reds. To get the best antioxidant concentrations, keep an eye out for:

1 *Age of wine*: wait for the grape skin to soak in the wine for a year or, preferably, five years.

2 *Kind of grape* (the *cépage*): the thicker the skin, the more the antioxidant load, hence the better for the health. Go for Merlot grape wines (found in St Emilion, Pomerol and Médoc wines), Cabernet Sauvignon (blended with Merlot for Pomerol and Médoc and Chilean wines), Syrah (found in Côte Rôtie and Australian Shiraz wines) and Sangiovese (found in Italian Tucson Chianti wine).

3 *Humidity*: wines grown in the humid regions, such as Burgundy, have developed natural antioxidant defenses against fungal attacks.

4 *Temperature*: grapes grown where they need more protection from the UV rays (hotter climates such as Chile, Portugal, southern France, Australia, California), will naturally develop more natural antioxidant

The best drinking pattern is daily red wine consumption with meals defenses that they can pass on to you. In particular, the antioxidant phenols (catechin and quercetin) is thought to have the ability to bind and eliminate (chelate) pro-oxidant metals that would be clogging your arteries.

In sum, it appears that the best drinking pattern is daily red wine consumption with meals. Red wine used in this way should be part of any therapy against the insidious diseases that plague us.

How to Order Wine in a Restaurant

If you do not have the good fortune of being a *maître sommelier*, rest assured. There are easy and effective ways to compensate for an incomplete understanding of the wines on the list:

1 *Take your time*: this is a time-honored ritual that just will not be rushed. This is genuinely fun. Of course, a little bit of research beforehand is well worth it in terms of helping to find a fine bottle or two to round out the meal and make it memorable. If you are planning to spend a significant amount of money (anniversaries, birthdays, important rendezvous), call ahead to the restaurant and have them fax you their wine list during the afternoon, to give you time to get online to help make the optimal choice.

2 *Don't be intimidated and feel free to experiment*: French wines are generally fine, but wines from Australia, California, Chile, Argentina, and South Africa can also be excellent. Wine is a learning experience of trial and error, not just a beverage.

3 *Get the wine list right away*: while you are scanning the wine list, begin with elegance by ordering an aperitif (Kir Royal or dry white wine).

4 *The opening ritual*: it is your pleasure to examine the label (the château, the year of bottling (the vintage), the producer and, of course, the type of wine):

   ■ **Start with the eyes** – check the cork to see if it is moist (a sign of being stored on its side to seal the wine from the air and light).

   ■ While the glass is on the table, swirl the glass to get the precious nectar to rise up on to the walls of the glass. **Check out the "legs"** of the wine – good legs indicate a higher alcohol content and thicker body.

■ **Move to the nose** – this gentle swirling also helps to get the bouquet airborne where your sense of smell can appreciate it. Pick up the glass by the foot (base) so as not to change the temperature of the wine. Raise the glass up to your nose and slowly insert your entire proboscis into the glass and inhale slowly and deeply. All eyes are on you, but you are deep in reverie, remembering the last romantic moment that such nectar flowed or imagining what the climatic conditions must have been and so on. But don't leave your dinner guests too long: do come back to the tasting.

■ **Move to the mouth** – as your nose has already tasted the wine, there should be few nasty surprises at this point. While puckering your lips, inhale so as to gently coax the wine over the respective taste buds in the mouth: sweet (at the tip), sour (at the sides), salty (on the flat surface) and bitter (at the back). Study the aftertaste as the wine parades through the mouth.

■ **Send it back** – if the wine appears in any way to be suboptimal (your tastebuds know, even if you cannot articulate it, any scent of cork or vinegar), you may send it back (it will be sold by the glass once properly exposed to air). No sweat at all. Whether you buy the bottle or not, remember the label and the year so as to build up your own database of "winners" for next time.

5 *Like with like*: obviously, you will already know what you like and how much you want to spend (your afternoon research will also prevent you from being overcharged). Your next step is to ask the other guests what type of entrées they will be having to synchronize the wine with the food:

■ **Red wine** – red wines have loads of tannin and flavor that would be well matched with game meat (boar, venison, pheasant), beef, lamb and pork.

■ **White wine** – generally well matched with chicken, poultry and fish. Fish is often cooked with lemon to enhance the flavor (which clashes with the flavor of red wine).

A Compassionate View on Alcoholism

Why is it that some people have a difficult time controlling alcohol in their lives? Is it genetic? Is it the alcohol? Are those people just hooked? In the interest of developing a more compassionate view of friends and colleagues who might be alcoholics, several meaningful insights can be gleaned from some excerpts from the historic 1961 letters between Bill Wilson, one of the co-founders of Alcoholics Anonymous, and Carl Jung.[5] They are discussing a patient of Jung's, Roland H., a resistant alcoholic:

Bill Wilson: *My recollection of his [Roland H's] account of that conversation is this: First of all, you frankly told him of his hopelessness, so far as any further medical or psychiatric treatment might be concerned. This candid and humble statement of yours was beyond doubt the first foundation stone upon which our Society has since been built. Coming from you, one he so trusted and admired, the impact was immense.*

When he then asked you if there was any other hope, you told him that there might be, provided he could become a subject of a spiritual or religious experience – in short, a genuine conversion …

This book [William James' Varieties of Religious Experience*] gave me the realization that most conversion experiences, whatever their variety, do have a common denominator of ego collapse at depth. The individual faces an impossible dilemma …*

In the wake of my spiritual experience, there came a vision of a society of alcoholics, each identifying with and transmitting to the next – chain style. If each sufferer were to carry the news of the scientific hopelessness of alcoholism to each new prospect, he might be able to lay every newcomer wide open to a transforming spiritual experience. This concept proved to be the foundation of such success as Alcoholics Anonymous has since achieved. This has made conversion experiences – nearly every variety reported by James – available on almost a wholesale basis …

Very many thoughtful AAs are students of your writings. Because of your conviction that man is something more than intellect, emotion and two dollars' worth of chemicals, you have especially endeared yourself to us …

Please be certain that your place in the affection, and in the history, of our Fellowship is like no other.

Gratefully yours,

William G. Wilson

Carl Jung: *… His [Roland H's] craving for alcohol was the equivalent, on a low level, of the spiritual thirst of our being for wholeness; expressed in medieval language: the union with God.*

How could one formulate such an insight in a language that is not misunderstood in our days?

The only right and legitimate way to such an experience is that it happens to you in reality, and it can only happen to you when you walk a path that leads to higher understanding. You might be led to that goal by an act of grace or through a personal and honest contact with friends, or through a higher education of the mind beyond the confines of mere rationalism....

I am strongly convinced that the evil principle prevailing in this world leads the unrecognized spiritual need into perdition if it is not counteracted either by religious insight or by the protective wall of the human community. An ordinary man, not protected by an action from above and isolated in society, cannot resist the power of evil, which is aptly called the Devil ...

You see, "alcohol" in Latin is spiritus, *and we use the same word for the highest experience as well as the most depraving poison. The helpful formula therefore is* spiritus contra spiritum.

Thanking you again for your kind letter,

I remain

yours sincerely

C.G. Jung

The Immune System as a Radar System

Fig. 3.1 (page 78) shows the different stages whereby cancer can manifest itself in the human body.

To avoid inviting cancer into your life:

1 Increase your internal resistance:
   - activity – disease hates moving targets!
   - optimize body fat (< 20% for men, < 23% women) – walk away from cancer!
   - sleep – pay all REM (rapid eye movement sleep) debts this month
   - mind control – accept delivery of only positive thoughts
   - control negativism in your life – laugh heartily every day!

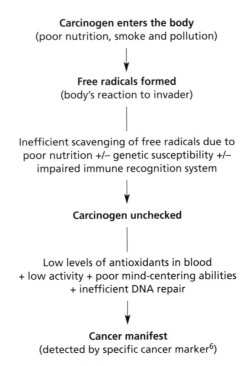

Carcinogen enters the body
(poor nutrition, smoke and pollution)

Free radicals formed
(body's reaction to invader)

Inefficient scavenging of free radicals due to
poor nutrition +/– genetic susceptibility +/–
impaired immune recognition system

Carcinogen unchecked

Low levels of antioxidants in blood
+ low activity + poor mind-centering abilities
+ inefficient DNA repair

Cancer manifest
(detected by specific cancer marker[6])

FIGURE 3.1 *The immune system as a radar system*

2 Decrease external carcinogens:

- no cigarettes
- no fried foods
- no sugars.

3 Get checked out from time to time:

- testicles and prostate for men
- breast, cervix and ovaries for women.

Detoxify the Body with Antioxidants

Cheap Health Insurance or Expensive Urine?

The problem of premature aging and disease is an uncontrolled oxidative process.[7] The oxidative process has been described by molecular biologists as an integral element of a Unifying Theory of Health. This theory incriminates oxygen-induced compounds known as *free radicals* as causative agents in seemingly unrelated degenerative diseases such as heart disease, cancers, autoimmune diseases, diabetes, arthritis and premature aging.

So, what are free radicals? Free radicals that do manage to escape the normal defenses of the body (up to 5%) damage the cells of the body at the molecular level, eroding the body's natural defenses and increasing our susceptibility to heart disease, cancers and other insidious diseases. Free radicals are, in essence, unpaired (unstable) electrons in a world where stability and homeostasis want paired electrons (see Fig. 3.2).

The problem of premature aging and disease is an uncontrolled oxidative process

$$- C - C - C - C - C - C - C -$$

FIGURE 3.2 *A molecule with an unpaired electron (free radical)*

Although millions of free radicals are produced as the normal metabolic and chemical processes take place every day, there are two ways in which we can decrease their negative effects:

- avoiding generating new free radicals (sources of free radicals include UV radiation and pollution – including cigarette smoke, frying, and especially deep-frying, foods);
- taking in our nutrition the critical elements (the antioxidants) that can scavenge those free radicals that escape the body's normal defenses.

Antioxidants[8] benefit the health in a number of different ways:

- They stabilize the destruction of cells through neutralization of the free radicals that initiate and promote tumor growth.
- Substantial data from animal and human research models suggest that antioxidants block the process of arteriosclerosis (by blocking the oxidation of LDL cholesterol, an important step in plaque build-up in the cells of the arteries, eventually leading to heart attacks and strokes). These powerful allies in health work by blocking this detrimental process of oxidation.[9]
- Compelling evidence indicates that a diet low in antioxidants (e.g. Vitamin C, A and E, beta-carotene, selenium) increases the probability of developing cancers such as lung, breast and prostate. The mechanism involves blocking free radicals and polycyclic aromatic hydrocarbons from damaging DNA.

Getting Detoxified Naturally

There are other ways to develop an antioxidant strategy if you are a non-drinker. This is one of the major debates in nutritional medicine these days: whether we can get adequate amounts of essential nutrients from our food chain. Widespread consumer mistrust has resulted from revelations of noxious additives found in our foods: e.g. antibiotics and growth hormones.

Vitamin E (Tocopherol)

■ **Mechanism of action**: shown to block the oxidative modification of LDL (a 10-year follow-up in a large nurses' health study revealed that Vitamin E was associated with a 34% drop in heart disease), also delays aging of the brain and immune system by prolonging the life of the cells by blocking oxidative damage to band-3 proteins (strands of special proteins found in mammalian brains and the immune system). In a recent study of 30,000 male smokers in Finland between 50 and 70, researchers found that a 50 mg dose of synthetic Vitamin E taken for five to eight years lowered the incidence of prostate cancer by over 30%, and decreased deaths from prostate cancers by 41%.
■ **Found naturally in**: cold-press vegetable oils, fish oils, eggs, organ meats, molasses, seeds, nuts, wheat germ and avocados.

Vitamin C (Ascorbic acid/calcium ascorbate)

■ **Mechanism of action**: helps in wound healing, iron absorption, and red blood cell formation. Ascorbic acid is also an extremely powerful antioxidant.
■ **Found naturally in**: bell peppers, kiwis, spinach, lemons, kiwis, citrus fruits (oranges, grapefruit) and broccoli.

Beta-carotene (precursor to Vitamin A)

■ **Mechanism of action**: by neutralizing free radicals, it lowers the risk for cancers and heart disease (by 50%) in those with the pre-existing disease state.[10]
■ **Found naturally in**: carrots (25 mg, a therapeutically effective dose, is found in two large carrots), green cabbage, spinach, cantaloupe, broccoli and fruits.

Selenium

- **Mechanism of action**: there are several forms of this soil-based trace mineral, of which the most powerful is methylselenol. It is essential in the enzyme activities of antioxidants and has an ability to kill cancer cells themselves while inhibiting the growth of blood vessels that feed tumors; it shows particular promise against breast, colon and prostate cancer. It is very toxic at dosages of 100 *micro*grams.
- **Found naturally in**: mushrooms, meat, tuna, herring, sesame seeds, poultry, grains, nuts, garlic and eggs.

Lycopene

- **Mechanism of action**: lowers risk of prostate and colon cancer.
- **Found naturally in**: red cabbage and tomatoes.

Isothiocyantes

- **Mechanism of action**: protects against lung and prostate cancers.
- **Found naturally in**: broccoli (Number 1 Cancer Buster, according to the American National Cancer Institute), apples and strawberries.

Polyphenols

- **Mechanism of action**: raises HDL, lowers LDL (bad) cholesterol. Quercetin and catechin have demonstrated powerful protective effects against fat oxidation, a process leading to artery clogging.
- **Found naturally in**: red wine.

Cleaning oils

- **Mechanism of action**: in a large-scale clinical trial organized by the Italian National Association of Hospital Cardiologists it was demonstrated that adding just one gram of omega-3 fatty acid daily to other lifestyle recommendations could lower the risk of death after a heart attack by 20%.
- **Found naturally in**: salmon, trout, mackerel, sardines and Chinese water snake oil (EPA/DHA). Take one tablespoon/day of each oil, found in flax, hemp, safflower, sunflower, soybean, pumpkin and sesame oils (LA/LNA). Take at the same time as other supplements.

Niacin (B3)[11]

- **Mechanism of action**: niacin lowers LDL and slows the release of fatty acids from fat cells, thereby lowering the TGs.

Getting Detoxified with Help from Supplements

It is also possible to develop an antioxidant statedgy using supplements as follows:

- **Vitamin E**: 400–1200 IU (1.50 IU of Vitamin E = 1 mg) daily (with the heaviest meal).
- **Ascorbic acid/Calcium ascorbate**: 3–4 gr/day (crystals are more efficiently absorbed). This is a well-researched antioxidant to help repair micro-damage to tissues caused by smoking, pollution or stress.
- **Beta-carotene**: 25,000 IU/day (10 IU of beta-carotene = 1 mg retinol) (with breakfast).
- **Selenium**: 250 *micro*grams/day.
- **Essential oils** :
  - LA/ LNA: One tablespoon/day of each oil, found in flax, hemp, safflower, sunflower, soybean, pumpkin and sesame oils. Take at the same time as other supplements.
- **Cleaning oils**:
  - EPA/DHA: found in salmon, trout, mackerel, sardines and Chinese water snake oil.
- **Niacin (B$_3$)**: if your LDL stays high (> 1.60 g/l), if your TGs stay high (> 1.40 g/l) or your HDL stays low (> 0.45 g/l), try niacin: 100 mg + aspirin (30 mg) with dinner. Monitor blood glucose.

The Secret Garden of Sleep

It is altogether appropriate that the topic of sleep be dealt with in a chapter on wine, as they are often intimately involved. But what happens during sleep, an activity that occupies a full one third of our earthly existence, more than any other singular activity? What happens if we do not furnish enough rest for the mind and body? And what is the function of dreams and nightmares?

The Sleep Cycle

The sleep cycle is a sort of journey, made by the mind, in its innate wisdom, in search of not just rest from the day's events, but also a way to process everything that was too traumatic or difficult to cope with on the spot. Sleep, therefore, represents a unique opportunity to explore our inner selves, and our bedroom is the threshold. We depart on this journey, passing through alternating phases of sleep. The first phase is called NREM (non-rapid eye movement) sleep, and is composed of four stages of increasing stupor. Stages 3 and 4 are the deepest stages of stupor, during which we undergo the strongest experience of subjective sleep, known as slow wave sleep (SWS). At the end of each NREM phase (about 90–120 minutes), we come up out of the depths and enter a very special realm called paradoxical or REM[12] sleep.

Sleep represents a unique opportunity to explore our inner selves

There are separate functions of NREM and REM sleep. During NREM, we repair and regenerate various components of a fatigued body, which is why we sleep so well after a physically active day. To achieve this process of rejuvenation, the brain orders more cell repair through active cell division, energy is conserved, oxygen consumption slows and the secretion of more growth hormone[13] takes place. Every system in the body, with the exception of the brain and spinal cord, regenerates itself on a continuous basis, so much so that we are never the same person that we were several months ago. Thus, NREM = *body maintenance and repair.*

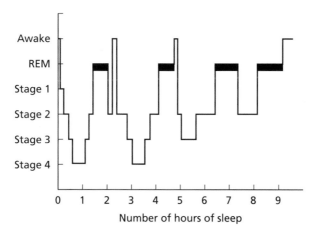

FIGURE 3.3 *The sleep cycle*

The REM stage, on the other hand, takes care of *mind maintenance*. REM sleep is in charge of dreaming, processing those events that were too difficult to deal with immediately during the day and, therefore, have been repressed into our subconscious. During REM (on *our own* terms and in the compressed time scale of dreaming) we process events of the day and file them into the respective thought files and memory banks of the mind (see Chapter 6 for a discussion on the brain). As infants are relative newcomers to the whole game of life and learning, it is not surprising that they spend more than twice the amount of sleeping time in REM (more unprecedented events to file into the memory). The more traumatic or stressful events that occur during the day, the greater the need for REM sleep, otherwise there will be a backlog of events to process – REM debt (a loss of REM sleep that accumulates from one night to the next). The results of a REM debt are predictable: decline in short-term memory and judgement, poorer attention, poorer communication, more irritability, more depression and less productivity.

> The biggest problem with REM-deprived people is that they are unaware of their impairment.

Dreams

Freud, in his *Interpretation of Dreams*, thought that dreams were a "royal road" to the deeper understanding of our psyche. Critical information, coming into our lives through the stream of positive and negative life events, must be converted into lessons regularly, otherwise a backlog occurs, particularly if the REM phases of sleep are repressed.

The third-century Taoist, Chang Tsu, once dreamed so vividly that he was a butterfly that he awoke (clearly during REM) exclaiming, 'Did Chang Tsu dream he was a butterfly or did the butterfly dream that it was Chang Tsu?"

If they are not dealt with, deferred thoughts will result in insomnia (the consciousness is struggling with the backlog), nightmares, depression and psychosomatic symptoms (headaches, ulcers, psoriasis, sleeplessness, asthma, panic attacks and, ultimately, illness). Moreover, dreams are the memory-processing phase when stored information can be reprocessed during REM, including memory necessary for survival.

Optimizing Your REM Sleep

What if we do not get enough REM? Though there is wide variation between people, on average the human adult requires a solid 8–9 hours to get enough REM to process the day's events. However, in our headlong rush since the Industrial Revolution towards the 24-hour culture, we have been losing an average of 1.5 hours per night of valuable sleep, or a total annual loss of about 550 hours of sleep! The symptoms of a civilization that is chronically tired are clear every day upon cursory inspection of the newspapers: errors in judgement while driving or flying, irritability, road rage, depression and, eventually, illness (see Fig. 3.4).

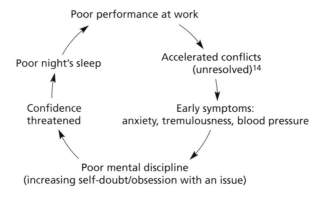

FIGURE 3.4 *Vicious circle of sleep (REM) deprivation*

Recent studies have shown that chronic fatigue can hinder proper motor and cerebral function as much as, if not more than, the effect of alcohol. In 1997, researchers published a ground-breaking study[15] wherein the loss of performance due to fatigue was quantified and compared to alcohol's impairment. The results were eye-opening: when kept awake for stretches of 18–27 hours, simple test performance deteriorated to an equivalent of a blood alcohol level (BAL) of more than 0.05%. An entire day without the benefits of sleep was equivalent to a BAL of 0.096, well above the legal limit in most countries.

You cannot buy REM sleep, nor induce more, but REM happens quite naturally when we allow it. Here are five steps to optimizing REM:

1 *Pay the REM debt*: recent studies have inferred that inadequate sleep quality can reduce the effectiveness of your immune system, making you an easy target for colds and flu and, possibly, cancer long-term. A stressful job, family conflicts, traveling and living in hotels, can *all* have

a major influence on the quality of your sleep. **Important health note**: avoid sleeping pills, caffeine products and alcohol prior to sleeping; they can cut out REM sleep.

2 *Calm the ambience*: here are some ways to calm the ambience in preparation for the night's rest:

- Use your bedroom as a sanctuary, a refuge: reserved for love and rest. *No* financial discussions, or marital discord. If you need to quarrel, leave the sanctuary (you would not argue in a temple, church or synagogue). Restrict the argument to the den or kitchen, in calm silence, out of earshot of the children. Never argue or create negative emotions that will possibly overwhelm your REM.
- Eat a light dinner and consume alcohol moderately. If you had a heavy business dinner, go for a 20-minute walk to start consuming the calories ingested. Lie on your right side (the side your stomach empties on).
- Move the TV out of the bedroom.
- Massage: the laying on of hands has a tremendous healing power.
- Love-making.

3 *Fatigue the body*: there are a number of ways to fatigue the body in preparation for the night's rest:

- Exercise, when optimally performed 4 hours before bedtime, can improve sleep quality.
- Burn the adrenaline, through a 4-minute workout.
- Drink warm (whole) milk with a spoon of honey. *Note*: caffeine, with a half-life of approximately 5 hours, should not be consumed after 2 pm.

4 *Calm the mind*: there are several ways to calm the mind in preparation for the night's rest:

- Bathing (floating): a warm bath will help to transform you gently from Type A (aggressive) to Type B (relaxed) person.
- Humor: particularly if it results in cheek cramps and tears.
- Deep breathing.
- Reading non-technical literature.
- Visualization.
- Do not overload the REM system: tie up any loose ends.
- Let go of anger: never go to bed angry.

5 *Progressive muscular relaxation* (PMR):[16] focus your attention on your head, relax your facial muscles and your jaws. Do *not* squeeze your teeth together. Relax your mouth and your lips and open your mouth slightly. Relax your neck and shoulder muscles. Visualize, while exhaling your breath, that you are exhaling all the tension of your body. Relax your arms, your hands and your fingers. Let go of all the tension like a wave movement. Relax your chest, your abdomen muscles, your buttocks. Now focus your attention on your legs: relax your thighs, your knees, your feet, ankles and toes. Just let go of it all.

Now bring your attention to your spine. Starting from the neck, let your focus slowly travel down the entire length of the spine to the lowest vertebra. As you let go and relax, notice that your entire back is relaxing, it is free of tension and feeling warm and comfortable. Now that your entire body is totally relaxed and free of tension, your blood can circulate more freely.

Focus your attention on your breathing and exhale all the remaining tension of your mind. Allow yourself to disengage, like taking your car out of gear. Disengage and listen to the silence of your mind. Breathe in deeply, relax, breathe out all the tension of your mind. Don't let your thoughts disturb your peaceful night, let them pass and allow yourself to switch off completely.

You are going to sleep deeply and free of all thoughts. You feel relaxed and serene. Visualize sleeping as a healing process. You are going to heal your body and your mind with a well-deserved good night's sleep … A warm night is waiting for you.

Just relax and let go … let go of all the tension of your body and your mind … Don't think; just let go and let yourself be pulled in by your dreams. Enter the fantasy world of your dreams in a totally relaxed state … Have a good night's sleep.

Preparing Meals

When it comes to preparing a meal for friends and family, these are only a few absolutes, as follows:

- In general, it is preferable, whenever possible, to cook together with a loved one while chatting about the day's events and listening (and humming) to soft background music with a glass of wine.

Never rush the preparation of a meal!

- Never rush the preparation of a meal! That defeats the whole purpose: a meal in France is a pleasure, starting from mincing garlic to sipping the Armagnac. Fine dining with loved ones is one of the reasons for working hard.
- Use *fresh* ingredients: nothing canned or stale.
- Lastly, your meal is your offering of love to your friends and family. Keep this in mind while cooking.

Breakfast

Breakfast is a very important meal. After all, you have been fasting all night long, while maintaining a high metabolic rate by engaging in plenty of REM fantasies and dreams. You will not see a great variety of recipes for breakfast because it is a meal with little time to prepare. However, it is a meal when we should strive to get the daily dose of roughage or fiber into the system.

The choices:

1 The *juices*: best choices include any fruit juice that has *no* added sugar (check the label) and has retained the pulp or fiber: carrots, apples, kiwi, grapefruit, or tomato. Fruit-flavored drinks made from concentrates are only slightly better than commercial soft drinks.

2 The *breads*: best choices include any breads that fill you up with whole grains or seeds (sunflower, poppy, sesame), such as those found in German bakeries: dark moist breads, covered with seeds.

3 The *sugars*: you need energy from a variety of sources, but not from refined sugars. If your body fat is greater than 5%, you have adequate stores without resorting to refined sugars such as those found in pastries.

4 The *proteins*: best choices include two poached/boiled free-range eggs, with grilled tomatoes (and beans, as optional), or *omelet d'Orvanne* (cheese, avocados).

5 The *fats*: best choices include any fats that are not excessively saturated. The fats commonly found on breakfast tables in order of decreasing benefit (i.e. best first) are fatty fish (herring, mackerel, salmon), beef, pork, bacon, lard.

For optimal health and energy, here are some breakfast suggestions for the heart and palate:

- Fresh blended kiwi juice, jasmine tea, whole wheat toasts with fresh butter and homemade jam.

- Cottage cheese or fromage blanc with fresh pineapple, Earl Grey tea with raisin or rye toast.
- Fresh pineapple juice, whole wheat cereals with fresh yoghurt and fruits, green tea.
- Freshly squeezed orange juice, green tea and whole wheat rye bread with fresh butter and homemade apple spread.
- Fresh apple juice, big fruit salad with green or jasmine tea.
- Poached eggs with grilled tomatoes and mushrooms. Whole wheat toasts with fresh butter, tea and fresh juice.
- Cheese, onion, tomato and omelette. Whole wheat rye with fresh butter, tea and freshly squeezed fruit juice.
- Whole wheat or rye bread with butter, coffee or tea without sugar.
- Yoghurt with non-acid fresh fruits, coffee or tea without sugar.
- Freshly squeezed orange juice and fresh fruit salad.
- Whole wheat cereal with yoghurt, banana and raisin.

Snacks and Miscellaneous

Some choices:

- Humus.
- Tarama.
- Homemade mayonnaise: place an egg yolk (separated from the egg white) in a bowl and, using a whisk, whip into the egg yolk a teaspoon of Dijon mustard. Continue the whisking while starting to drip in olive oil. You know if it is going to work if you see "strings" appear in the mixture as you drip in the oil. The best mayonnaise is made from a mixture of oils (sunflower, olive and hemp).

Lunch and Dinner (Fish and Seafood)

If you *cannot* walk afterwards, these options are optimal:

- Roasted chicken with green peas.
- Leg of lamb with beans.
- Onion and mushroom omelette.
- Fish or seafood or steak (rare) with vegetables.

If you *can* walk afterwards, these options are fine:

- Pasta cooked with olive oil, garlic and fresh tomatoes.
- Wild rice with onions and mushrooms.
- Potato stew with green beans, onions and tomatoes.
- Vegetable soup with garlic bread.

TIPS FOR YOUR HEALTH ACTION PLAN

The best blood thinners ... aspirin, red wine, EPA/DHA, garlic and onions, flax, hemp oil, apples, cherries, carrots

The best juices ... kiwi, carrot + pineapple, carrot + ginger + celery

The best sleep inducers ... whole milk (warmed) with honey

The best cooking oil ... olive, palm, ghee (clarified butter)

The best cancer buster ... broccoli, carrot

The best eating oil ... hemp, flax, olive, safflower

The best alcoholic drink ... red wine

The best non-alcoholic drink ... water, kiwi juice, fresh lime/lemon juice (without sugar), tomato/carrot juice

The best fat-burning exercise ... brisk walking after meal

The best hotel workout ... yoga, skipping rope, 4-minute workout

The best snack ... nut mix (especially almonds, cashews and sunflower seeds), fresh fruits (kiwi, apple and cherries)

The best hors d'oeuvres ... olives (black, green or stuffed), humus, cherry tomatoes, guacamole, raw carrots with homemade mayonnaise

Frequently Asked Questions

Alcohol and Health

Q Beer? Whiskey? White wine?

- **Beer**: beer (and malt whiskies) contains maltose (the sugar from malt), which has a Glycemic Index of 150, which causes insulin to surge. In a word, beer makes us fat, particularly around the waistline. Grapes have a Glycemic Index of only 66, which causes a very low insulin surge. In a word, drinking wine makes you thin.

In a study by the Institut National pour la Santé et la Recherche Médicale (INSERM) in Bordeaux, designed to see whether beer protects the heart from heart attacks, researchers found that those middle-aged men who drank two to five glasses of wine a day had a 29–33% lower death rate over abstainers. Beer drinkers had no such reduction in death rates, although both wine and beer drinkers had lower rates from heart disease and stroke. Cheers!

■ **Whiskey**: Slàinte! The word whiskey (from the Gaelic *uisge beatha*, for "water of life") for the Americans, and the Irish or whisky for the Scots, has overseen many critical political or economic decisions. The real issue at hand is the presence of toxins (fusel oil, which is almost pure amyl alcohol), impurities, carcinogens and depressants in the various distilled alcohol preparations. Alcohol distilled from potatoes has the highest amount of fusel oil, followed by alcohols distilled from grains and then grapes.

■ **White wine:** the protective antioxidant components of red wine are the polyphenol group (which includes quercetin, anthocyanidins and catechins), which make up, by weight, about 80% of the total phenols found in red wine. Lacking the source of these valuable antioxidants (the skin of the red grape), white wine has six times less phenols than red wines.

Final note: wine drinkers tend to sip their drink slowly with food, while beer drinkers tend to drink beer very rapidly outside meals.

Q Is it best **not to drink** at all?

■ While heavy drinking (more than 6 drinks a day) causes blood pressure to rise, up to three drinks a day is associated with reduced coronary heart disease. Studies have shown the relative risk of dying (mostly from coronary disease) to be 38% higher among non-drinkers compared to responsible drinkers. Cheers!

Q As a Chinese manager living in Hong Kong, I have been struck by the differences in **alcohol tolerance** (the facial redness) between my Western colleagues and myself. Why is this?

■ This flush reaction that happens to Asians (Japanese, and Chinese) and non-Asians (American Indians) is due to the higher levels of acetaldehyde (a toxin) and a lack of a special enzyme (aldehyde dehydrogenase – ALDH). However, in a Swedish study there emerged a syndrome known as "alcohol allergy," which included a constellation of asthma, skin swelling, nausea, and fainting present in up to 4.5% of all subjects.

Q What are the other health benefits of **aspirin** aside from blood thinning?

■ The Physicians' Health Study[10] put aspirin on the health map in a big way, demonstrating a 33% drop in non-fatal heart attacks in those doctors over 50 years of age. Aspirin (acetyl salicylic acid: 50 mg is as effective as 350 mg – without side effects) makes the blood thin, lowers fever, relieves pain and decreases inflammation. Recently published data have demonstrated the central role of aspirin in preventing the development of certain cancers (colon).

Q Are **onions and garlic** indispensable as part of the Mediterranean diet?

■ Yes. Onions and garlic decrease the production of cholesterol, help restore elasticity to the arteries, and make the blood thinner by decreasing platelet stickiness. Moreover, garlic acts to rid the body of toxins.

Q When I use alcohol (red wine and occasional spirits), I often awake a little **groggy**. Is this a hangover?

■ Alcohol has many effects on the sleep cycle:
  – after transient sedation, it can arouse certain sensitive individuals;
  – it increases snoring and sleep apnea;[15]
  – it diureses (causes urination) both water and minerals (calcium, magnesium, and potassium).

Q What is a **hangover** (*gueule de bois*)?

■ Hangovers are caused by a constellation of metabolic problems including dehydration, low blood sugar and a build-up of metabolic poisons. There are two metabolic pathways for alcohol (ethanol), which could account for the symptoms of a hangover.
  The most commonly accepted pathway:

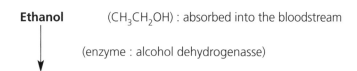

Ethanol   (CH_3CH_2OH) : absorbed into the bloodstream

(enzyme : alcohol dehydrogenasse)

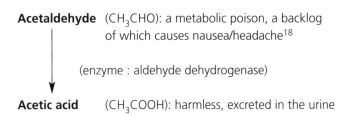

Acetaldehyde (CH_3CHO): a metabolic poison, a backlog of which causes nausea/headache[18]

(enzyme : aldehyde dehydrogenase)

Acetic acid (CH_3COOH): harmless, excreted in the urine

Another pathway, less commonly implicated in the symptoms:

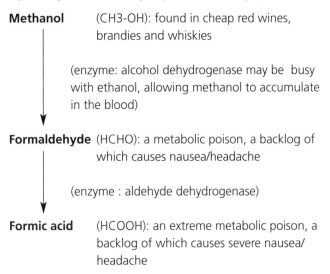

Methanol ($CH3-OH$): found in cheap red wines, brandies and whiskies

(enzyme: alcohol dehydrogenase may be busy with ethanol, allowing methanol to accumulate in the blood)

Formaldehyde ($HCHO$): a metabolic poison, a backlog of which causes nausea/headache

(enzyme : aldehyde dehydrogenase)

Formic acid ($HCOOH$): an extreme metabolic poison, a backlog of which causes severe nausea/ headache

Q How to **avoid a hangover**?

■ Compensate – avoid dehydration:
  - avoid drinking on an empty stomach, start with fruit juice or olives;
  - during drinking evenings, alternate alcohol with fruit juices;
  - before sleep, compensate water/mineral losses, take aspirin and sleep on your right side, the side your stomach empties on;
  - watch the old "1-2-3- punch": chips, fatty snacks, alcohol, coffee cycle.

Q Thickened blood: how did it happen and how can I thin the blood?

■ According to recent studies, thickened blood could increase the risks of strokes and heart attacks if blood-clotting factors (especially VW Factor, Factor VIIIc and fibrinogen) are activated. Obesity (excessive body fat), smoking, high BP, high TGs, and diabetes all thicken the blood, while exercise, stress management, smoking cessation and proper intake of the fat family all thin the blood.

Q If I have a body fat of 28%, a triglyceride level of 2.50 g/l and an HDL of 0.35 g/l, should I have the **occasional glass of wine** or not?

■ Get body fat into the 15% range by walking after meals for 15 minutes, Avoid all high Glycemic Index foods, while taking one glass of red wine slowly in the evenings for a month. Re-check your lab tests (TC, TGs and HDL) – you will be pleasantly surprised. Adjust the red wine intake according to the results, not exceeding three glasses per day (more alcohol than that may actually *increase* the TGs).

Q Women, **menopause** and alcohol?

■ Women who drink alcohol at a reasonable rate could be putting off their menopause, according to a two-year study of more than a thousand women aged 45–49. Of the women who drank no alcohol, 25% had reached the menopause, while only 6% of the women who drank one drink or more per day had reached it. The mechanism may be the estrogens boosting influences of alcohol.

Q What causes **heartburn** (stomach acidity refluxing into the esophagus)?

■ Consuming mints, chocolate, alcohol, wearing tight-fitting clothes and lying down within an hour of your meal.

Antioxidants and Other Supplements

Q What are some of the benefits of antioxidant **Vitamin C**?

■ Vitamin C (ascorbic acid) has well-documented antioxidant effects. For example, strokes are the result of a build-up of fatty deposits in arteries. This build-up is prevented by antioxidants, throughout the body.

Q We enjoy the occasional fried dishes (fish and chips). What are the **best oils** to do this in?

■ Excessively high heat that comes with frying is one way to introduce billions of dangerous free radicals into the body, particularly for the refined healthful oils (EFAs and polyunsaturated oils). In fact, saturated fats (like butter), though less healthful in general, are more stable against high temperatures, which brings us back to the French paradox once again. Alternatively, do as the traditional Chinese do and start by adding a bit of water into the pan or with the vegetables before adding the oil (which should be the more stable mono-unsaturated sort (olive) or tropical oils (coconut, palm, cocoa butter), peanut or sesame).

Sleep and Health

Q Is there a relationship between sleeping disorders and **high blood pressure**?

■ A new study by the American Lung Association confirmed that people with sleep-related breathing disorders (a condition in which the throat narrows repetitively throughout sleep producing snoring) are at increased risk of high blood pressure and heart disease.

Q Is there a relationship between sleep quality and the **menopause**?

■ Yes. Certain patients find relief from the hormonal imbalances through the use of naturopathic remedies such as evening primrose oil, hypericum and dong quai, supplemented by magnesium tablets at bedtime to relax the muscles.

Q Do other **animals** dream?

■ The normal sleep cycle, with alternating non-REM and REM sleep, is present in all mammals, both placental and marsupial. They exhibit the same kinds of various REM-type characteristics (such as EEG changes) as human beings, and these serve the same important survival functions.

SELF-ASSESSMENT QUIZ

1 Organic (disease) causes of fatigue:

   (a) Anemia
   (b) Cancer
   (c) Thyroid disease
   (d) Glandular fever

2 Functional (lifestyle) causes of fatigue:

   (a) Dehydration
   (b) Poor posture
   (c) Poor breathing
   (d) Low activity levels
   (e) Uncompensated stress
   (f) Poor sleep quality (low REM)

3 All alcohol has a beneficial effect on health:

(a) True
(b) False

Hint: HDL

4 Moderate consumption of alcohol (two to three glasses a day) can help prevent heart disease:

(a) True
(b) False

Hint: HDL

5 Red wine is more beneficial to the health than white wine, beer and spirits:

(a) True
(b) False

Hint: While all alcohols increase cardioprotective HDL, only red wine also thins blood

6 The brain is asleep when we are asleep:

(a) True
(b) False

Hint: During sleep (especially during REM), the brain processes (repressed) thoughts that we would not deal with during waking hours

7 Being sleepy is primarily due to boredom:

(a) True
(b) False

Hint: Sleepiness is due to low oxygen in the brain (poor breathing) and poor sleep quality (low REM)

8 Wine legs can tell you about:

(a) Year of bottling
(b) Body of the wine
(c) Alcohol content

9 REM backlogs: choose the correct statement:

(a) Are caused by sleeping medications and alcohol excess
(b) Can cause chronic fatigue

(c) Can be relieved by napping or meditation

Hint: Sleep hygiene is a quality, not quantity, issue!

10 Antioxidants can be obtained from foods naturally or by supplements:

(a) True
(b) False

Hint: The body's immune defenses recognize antioxidant assistance, either from natural foods or supplements

11 REM is for:

(a) Body maintenance
(b) Mind maintenance

12 Snoring is not harmful to the health, if no one is disturbed:

(a) True
(b) False

Hint: Snoring, often caused by obesity, can indicate poor oxygen supply to the brain

13 The best low Glycemic Index cocktail snacks include:

(a) Olives
(b) Nuts (peanuts, almonds)
(c) Crackers

Hint: Insulin stores fat

14 The best low Glycemic Index alcoholic drinks include:

(a) Wine
(b) Beer
(c) Champagne

Hint: Insulin stores fat

15 Which of the following suppresses REM?

(a) Alcohol
(b) Sleepers
(c) Sex
(d) Excessive stress

Answers

1 All	**6** (b)	**11** (b)
2 All	**7** (b)	**12** (b)
3 (a)	**8** (b) & (c)	**13** (a) & (b)
4 (a)	**9** All	**14** (a) & (c)
5 (a)	**10** (a)	**15** (a), (b) & (d)

Notes

1 What is meant by alcohol use is, of course, the use of ethyl alcohol or ethanol (C_2H_5OH).

2 See McKenna T., *Food of the Gods, The Search for the Original Tree of Knowledge*, (Bantam Books, 1992).

3 For decades health researchers have marveled how the French enjoy great longevity (see Chapter 1) despite their regular intake of fats and alcohol. Even a cursory inspection reveals the truth: there is no paradox at all – the high intake of red wine and walking infer a protective effect. Moreover, the French have (1) smaller portions of higher quality food (2) higher fruit and salad intake (3) regular eating hours (4) less money to spend on labor-saving devices, and, lastly (5) more respect for the body and the food going into it than most other cultures.

4 Facchini F. et al. "Light to moderate alcohol intake is associated with enhanced insulin sensitivity." *Diabetes Care*, 1994; 17: 115–18.

5 From the *Parabola Book of Healing,* Continuum Publishers,1994.

6 The various cancer markers are: prostatic specific antigen (PSA) and carcinoembrynoic antigen (CEA) for the intestine, alpha-fetoprotein (AFP) for the liver, ovaries and testes, and CA 27–29 for the breasts.

7 Oxidation: a normal body process in which reactive oxygen molecules – free radicals – play a destructive role by oxidizing LDL, damaging nucleic acids (in your DNA) and denaturing proteins. Therefore, antioxidation is the process of scavenging free radicals that cause accelerated tissue damage.

8 Antioxidants are one cornerstone of what is known as *orthomolecular medicine*, which refers to the supplementation of essential nutrients to enhance the internal defenses and resistance of the body.

9 A critical review of clinical trial data suggests that antioxidants (vitamin E, beta-carotene, and vitamin C) reduce cardiovascular disease by up to 65%, with the clearest effect for vitamin E. To achieve these reductions, supplementation of antioxidants must last for at least two years. See *Annals of Internal Medicine*. 1995; 123: 860–72.

10 The Physicians' Health Study, *New England Journal of Medicine,* 1989; 321: 129–35.

11 Niacin (B$_3$) protects our heart via two mechanisms: (1) when combined with Chromium, can lower cholesterol by up to 50% in patients with high levels, and (2) acts as an antioxidant against the toxic effects of oxidized adrenaline (adenochrome).

12 REM (rapid eye movement) sleep: vivid images in the form of dreams are flashed on the mind's screen. This causes the eyes, viewing this fantasy world, to dart to and fro, the blood pressure and heart rate increase, skin potential changes and the brain waves become more rapid, all as a function of the emotional make-up of our dreams. In a word, we are in a new reality.

13 As people age, they tend to get less slow wave sleep, which can cause a decrease in growth hormone. A recent study reveals that for middle-aged people who tend to gain weight this may be due to a lack of deep sleep, known as slow wave sleep. Growth hormone deficiencies have been associated with certain kinds of weight gain.

14 Clearly, in life no one can always avoid conflicts: they represent potential growth experiences, both personally and professionally. To convert this vicious sleep cycle into a virtuous sleep cycle, just make certain that every conflict is finished by a lesson. Otherwise, sleep will suffer and the life quality unravels.

15 *Nature*, 1997.

16 PMR (and other relaxation techniques) is available in CD form.

17 Sleep apnea refers to the phenomenon wherein alcohol-relaxing effects on the muscles of the upper airway cause the complete collapse of the throat, causing worsened snoring and, ultimately, breathing cessation (obstructive sleep apnea), especially in the obese.

18 The basis of this is the fact that a treatment for alcohol abuse is Antabuse (disulfiram), which blocks aldehyde dehydrogenase, an enzyme that causes the build-up of the poison acetaldehyde. It is estimated that a lack of aldehyde dehydrogenase occurs very commonly in Asians (estimated 50% of Japanese lack it), causing the common reaction to alcohol in Asians.

CHAPTER FOUR

WORKOUT

Doing as little as a 15-minute walk every day and a 4-minute workout every morning can dramatically transform your health and stamina, while decreasing your risk of premature death by more than 30%!

In the past even a duke had to do a lot of walking, even a money-lender, even a metaphysician. And when they weren't using their legs, they were jogging about on their horses. Whereas now, from the tycoon to the typist, from the logical positivist to the positive thinker, you spend nine tenths of your time sitting on foam rubber. Spongy seat for a spongy bottom – at home, in the office, in cars and bars, in planes, trains and buses. No moving of legs, no struggles with distances and gravity – just lifts and planes and cars, just foam rubber and an eternity of sitting. The life force that used to find its outlet through striped muscle gets turned back on the viscera and the nervous system and slowly destroys them.

ALDOUS HUXLEY, *ISLAND*

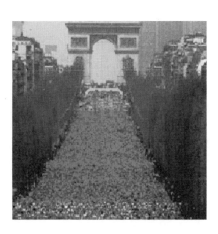

Using the advice contained in this chapter, Mr Timebomb could take care of the following health issues:

■ high cholesterol
■ high blood triglycerides
■ low HDL (good) cholesterol
■ low stamina
■ back pain
■ body fat.

Introduction

Every year many millions of dollars are expended on hospital admissions, medications, vitamins and health farms, while health and fitness seems to deteriorate. What has happened? What is necessary to keep all the balls in the air: a jog or a walk?

Our lifestyle has changed radically in the last 20 years, in complete discordance with our genetic code, our DNA. The model of the successful manager has significantly evolved since the days when a heart attack was considered just another part of the manager's territory. Today's executives have to develop ways to avail themselves of the traditional elements of success – dynamic balance, stamina, self-mastery and mental hardiness – while retaining optimal health. A regular physical workout takes care of all those success traits in one fell swoop.

The 4–Minute Workout

The following workout allows you to increase strength, endurance and stamina without a heavy investment in time. Three variations have been provided and you should select the appropriate one according to whether you are a beginner (Stage I), intermediate (Stage II) or advanced (Stage III).

You are a Stage I (beginner) if you:

■ have BP (blood pressure) > 160/100; or
■ have TG:HDL > 5; or
■ smoke > 20 cigarettes a day; or

- have LDL > 1.60 g/l; or
- BF (body fat) > 25%; or
- CF (cardiofitness) > 130 beats.

> Make best use of this highly effective workout and you will be "hard as a rock" within one month!

4-MINUTE WORKOUT FOR STAGE I ▶▶▶▶▶

Upon awakening, start to replace water losses that occurred during the night's sleep with a **glass of lemon/lime water** (room temperature water with a full lemon or lime squeezed into it). As the water settles, stand erect and **rub your palms together**, as if warming them vigorously, for 15 seconds.

1 Before actually starting your physical workout, **center the mind** in preparation for the day's stresses: either 1 minute of deep breathing, meditation or mantra will do, so choose according to your liking.

2 Next, **run in place** for 1 minute while breathing deeply, lifting the heels high enough to touch with your hands.

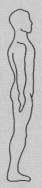 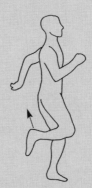

Have another glass of lemon/lime water.

3 Then, **stretch** to your left side for 15 seconds, followed by **stretch** to your right side for 15 seconds as shown below.

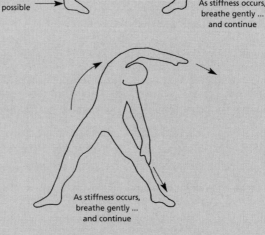

As wide as possible

As stiffness occurs, breathe gently ... and continue

As stiffness occurs, breathe gently ... and continue

4 Continue with 1 minute of **sink press-ups** against the sink or desk (at a 45–60° angle).

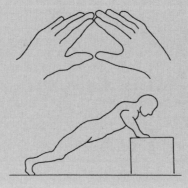

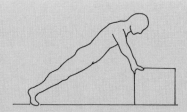

Have another glass of lemon/lime water.

5 Finish with 30 seconds of **curl-ups** (the "crunch"), exhaling every time you come up or strain. Use the sliding forward of the hands as an indicator of whether you are doing these correctly.

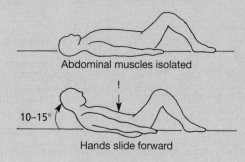

Abdominal muscles isolated

10–15°

Hands slide forward

Have another glass of lemon/lime water.

You are a Stage II (intermediate) if you:

- have BP 140/90–160/100; or
- have TG:HDL 3–5; or
- smoke < 20 cigarettes a day; or
- have LDL 1.30–1.60 g/l; or
- BF 20–25%; or
- CF = 100–130 beats.

4-MINUTE WORKOUT FOR STAGE II

Upon awakening, start to replace water losses that occurred during the night's sleep with a **glass of lemon/lime water** (room temperature water with a full lemon or lime squeezed into it). As the water settles, stand erect and **rub your palms together**, as if warming them vigorously, for 15 seconds.

1 Before actually starting your physical workout, **center the mind** in preparation for the day's stresses: either 30 seconds of deep breathing, meditation or mantra will do, so choose according to your liking.

2 Next, **jumping jacks** for 1 minute while breathing deeply, lifting the hands high enough to clap them overhead.

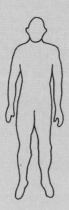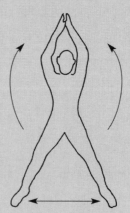

Have another glass of lemon/lime water.

3 Then, **stretch** to your left side for 15 seconds, followed by **stretch** to your right side for 15 seconds as shown below.

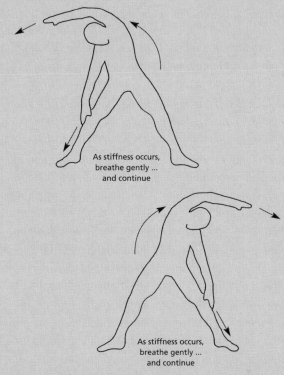

As stiffness occurs, breathe gently ... and continue

As stiffness occurs, breathe gently ... and continue

4 Continue with 30 seconds of **sink press-ups** against the sink or desk (at a 45–60° angle).

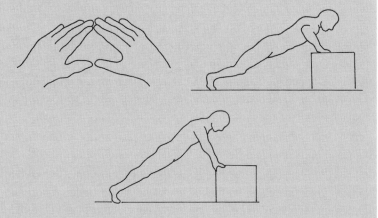

Have another glass of lemon/lime water.

5 Continue with 30 seconds of **chair dips**, exhaling every time you come up or strain.

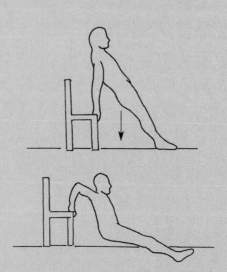

Have another glass of lemon/lime water.

6 Finish with 60 seconds of **curl-ups** (the "crunch"), exhaling every time you come up or strain. Use the sliding forward of the hands as an indicator of whether you are doing these correctly.

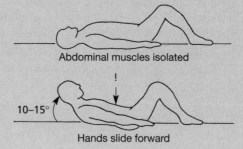

Abdominal muscles isolated

10–15°

Hands slide forward

You are in Stage III (advanced) if you:

- have BP < 140/90; and
- have TG: HDL < 3; and
- do not smoke cigarettes; and
- have LDL < 1.30 g/l; and
- BF < 20%; and
- CF < 100 beats.

4-MINUTE WORKOUT FOR STAGE III

Upon awakening, start to replace water losses that occurred during the night's sleep with a **glass of lemon/lime water** (room temperature water with a full lemon or lime squeezed into it). As the water settles, stand erect and **rub your palms together**, as if warming them vigorously, for 15 seconds.

1 Before actually starting your physical workout, **center the mind** in preparation for the day's stresses: either 30 seconds of meditation or mantra will do, so choose according to your liking.

2 Next, **jumping rope** for 1 minute while breathing deeply.

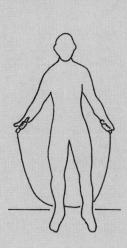
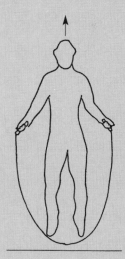

Have another glass of lemon/lime water.

3 Then, **stretch** to your left side for 15 seconds, followed by **stretch** to your right side for 15 seconds as shown below.

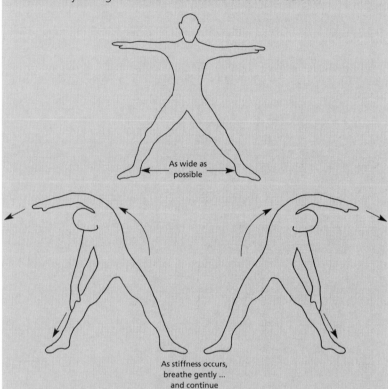

As wide as possible

As stiffness occurs, breathe gently ... and continue

4 Continue with 30 seconds of **spinal twist**.

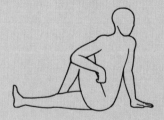

5 Continue with 30 seconds of **sink press-ups** against the sink or desk (at a 45–60° angle).

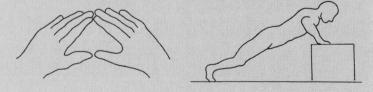

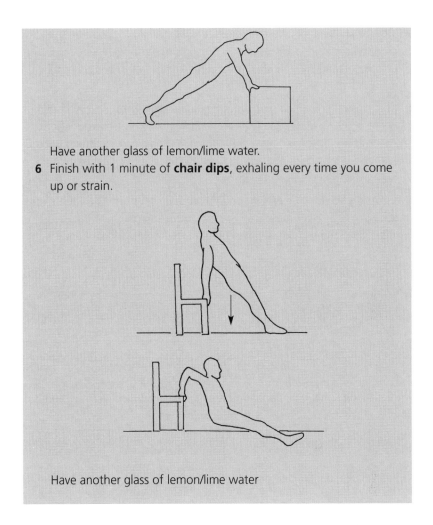

Have another glass of lemon/lime water.

6 Finish with 1 minute of **chair dips**, exhaling every time you come up or strain.

Have another glass of lemon/lime water

Instructions for the Exercises in the Various 4-Minute Workouts

Here is a more detailed explanation of how the exercises mentioned in the workouts should be performed:

■ **Running in place**: just run in place at the same rhythm and bounce as you would running on the beach or in the forest.

■ **Lateral stretch**: with bare feet spread as far as they can be comfortably and arms held out at sides, palms down, slide your right hand along your right thigh and lower leg until you hit a sticking point where it is difficult to go further. Breathe deeply and watch the muscles and tendons get more supple. Mentally mark the spot where your right hand was able to reach on your ankle. Come back up and repeat on left side.

- **Sink press-ups**: either with knees-bent or straight-legged, flat on ground or at 45°, perform the maximal number of push–ups (counting aloud) possible in 1 minute (no more!). Rest in the up position only, while breathing out on elevation.

- **Curl-ups** (the "crunch"): lift your head and shoulders off the ground about 15–20°, while sliding your hands along the floor towards your knees about 10 cms (4 inches). Perform the maximal number of curl-ups (counting aloud) possible in 1 minute (no more!). Rest in the up position only, while breathing out on elevation.

- **Jumping jacks**: with bare feet together, hold your arms at sides, palms down. When ready, jump up in air, smoothly spreading your feet just wider than the shoulders, while the arms form a full circle, gently touching over the head. As the legs help return blood to the heart, they represent a "second heart." Invest in them.

- **Chair dips**: using a chair (or any solid object of comparable height), keep your body straight and lower your buttocks to the ground, without resting them there, forming a right angle. Repeat for a 1-minute count (no more!).

In addition to the above exercises there is a great 30-second morning workout for toning your abdominal muscles that will also help to keep the intestines regular. It is called the **abdominal snap**. Breathing calmly and deeply, stand with knees slightly bent and the feet at the width of the shoulders, with the palms of the hands on the thighs, just above the knees. Slowly expel all the air from your lungs and then suck in your gut as far as possible. While still holding the breath gently, snap the gut out and repeat three times for that inhaled breath. This can tone the abdominal muscles while giving a "wake-up call" to otherwise lethargic intestines.

Practical Application

For those times when you are "on the road," traveling around the world, unable to fit in the workout necessary to condition your heart, we pro-pose a quick, but intense, 4-minute work-*ought* to be done every morning before going to work (see Table 4.1). This is a supplement to help you to get your blood oxygenated in the morning to build up your endurance in preparation for the day's stresses ahead of you. Perform I minute of each exercise as shown above. Fill in the chart opposite (with date) and add one more exercise jumping jacks, curl-ups, press-ups per day until you reach your *age* per minute (example: a 47 year old will do up to 47).

TABLE 4.1 *4-minute work*-ought

	Press–ups	Curl-ups	Chair dips	Jumping jacks	Jumping rope
Baseline (example)	12	34	10	3	30 sec.
Week One	**+1**	**+1**	**+1**	**+1**	**+10 sec.**
Monday					
Tuesday					
Wednesday					
Thursday					
Friday					
Saturday					
Sunday					
Week Two	**+3**	**+3**	**+3**	**+3**	**+20 sec.**
Monday					
Tuesday					
Wednesday					
Thursday					
Friday					
Saturday					
Sunday					
Week Three	**+10**	**+10**	**+10**	**+10**	**+30 sec.**
Monday					
Tuesday					
Wednesday					
Thursday					
Friday					
Saturday					
Sunday					
Week Four	**+10**	**+10**	**+10**	**+10**	**+60 sec.**
Monday					
Tuesday					
Wednesday					
Thursday					
Friday					
Saturday					
Sunday					

The Health Benefits of Working Out

There are many benefits of working out, both mental and physical

There are many benefits of working out, both mental and physical.

Mental Benefits

The mental benefits that can be gained from regular working out are listed below:

- feeling good or peaceful;
- better mental health (less depressive episodes);
- playfulness or communion with Nature/others;
- less loneliness;
- increased sexual satisfaction;[1]
- distraction from daily affairs;
- spiritual awakening of potential;
- preparing the body (the "temple") for meditation;
- improved self-confidence;
- better socialization skills;
- less anxiety;
- improved sexual expression;
- less symptoms of depression;
- better sleep;
- healthful distraction from "affairs";
- better preparedness for change;
- increased energy and stamina.

Physical Benefits

The physical benefits that can be achieved through regular exercise are equally as impressive:

- better physical health (inactive people have *six* times the risk of heart disease as active people);

- lowered heart rate and BP: determinants of heart muscle O_2 demand (drop is sustained for up to 12 hours);
- lowered total cholesterol (by up to 24%), LDL (up to 10%), triglycerides (fats);
- improved ability of artery linings to produce nitric oxide (relaxes arteries and makes them contract more efficiently);
- lowered body fat leads to lowered TG and LDL;
- increased HDL cholesterol (up to 6%);
- increased lean mass;
- increased work capacity;
- better lung function and gas exchange;
- feeling more energetic or feeling lighter;
- better joint flexibility, range of motion and bone mass;
- better strength and coordination;
- increased energy and stamina;
- better fat and sugar control;
- thinning of the blood (clotting reduced by 52%).

Protecting the Heart with FIT

We lose 1% of our cardiovascular efficiency (fitness) *per year*, if we do nothing about it. That is a full 40% by the time we reach the golden years at retirement age.

Regardless of your choice of exercise, to be of optimal effectiveness an exercise prescription for cardiovascular conditioning must adhere to these FIT guidelines:

F = Frequency: optimal frequency is three sessions a week or every other day.

I = Intensity: the training heart rate (THR): the steady-state heart beat.

T = Time: the duration of the exercise. Optimal = 20–30 minutes a session.

Steps to Calculate Your Training Heart Rate (THR)

Your THR is a "steady state" level of intensity that is both safe and effective in conditioning your heart. It is a percentage (65% would, general for example, be expressed as 0.65) of your maximal heart rate, calculated by the general formula below:

THR = [(220 – age – resting heart rate (RHR)) X intensity level] + RHR

Step 1: The intensity level is a function of your cardio-fitness rating

To determine your overall cardio-fitness level, you will need to perform the **step test**:

- make a step (newspapers or telephone books will do nicely) 30 cm (12") high;
- set a metronome at 96;
- step up and down on the step for 3 minutes at the rhythms dictated by the metronome. After 3 minutes of stepping, sit and find your pulse within 5 seconds;
- now carefully take your recuperating pulse for a *full minute* after stepping.

Using Table 4.2 you can then find the percentage corresponding to the fitness level you achieved. For example, if you are 46 and counted 124 beats in the first minute of recuperation, your level is "Below average," and your intensity is 0.65.

Step 2: Plug in all the variables in the formula

For example, a 46-year-old man, with an RHR of 72, intensity level of 0.65, would have a THR of: [(220 – 46 – 72) X 0.65] + 72 = 138 beats per minute.

So whatever activity this man has decided to do, in order to avail himself of the appropriate conditioning effects on the heart and mind, he should do that exercise for three sessions of 20 to 30 minutes a week at 138 beats/minute or 34 beats/15".

Ideally, you should always start your exercise for about 5 minutes, and then stop and check your pulse. If your measured THR is faster than the ideal, you're working too hard. If your pulse is slower than the ideal, pick up the pace until you reach your THR range.

TABLE 4.2 *How to determine your intensity level/cardio-fitness rating: the after-test heart rates for different age groups*

Level (Intensity)	Age 18–25	Age 26–35	Age 36–45	Age 46–55	Age 56–65	Age 65–99
Olympic (0.85)	up to 65	70	75	80	85	85
Athletic (0.80)	up to 75	80	85	90	95	100
Above average (0.75)	up to 90	95	95	100	110	115
Average (0.70)	up to 105	110	115	120	125	130
Below average. (0.65)	up to 125	130	135	140	145	150
Fair (0.60)	up to 150	160	140	160	170	175
Poor (0.55)	> 180	> 185	> 165	> 185	> 190	> 201

How shall I Progress Through the Various Stages of the FIT Program?

Once you have begun a conditioning program to strengthen the heart, you can move very smoothly through the conditioning stages in a few weeks. Here's how to progress safely.

As you work out regularly at your THR three times a week for 30 minutes per session, you will notice an improvement in the efficiency of your heart. Now you can monitor your progress yourself. No more working out "in the dark"! Every week, your resting heart rate and your step-test results will show the increasing efficiency of the cardiovascular system. For example, Table 4.3 shows what your trends will look like if your initial step test was 135 and your resting heart rate was 80.

Note: as the THR calculation is dependent on results from the step test and resting heart rate, as overall cardio-fitness improves, these figures will go down, while your training heart rate will go up.

Important health note: with regard to BP, moderate aerobics activity (55–70% of person's predicted maximal heart rate (MHR) performed 30–40 minutes five days a week) is recommended as the desired level of

TABLE 4.3 *Increasing efficiency of the cardiovascular system*

Week	Step test result	Resting heart rate
1	135	80
5	130	75
10	125	70
20	115	60
30	105	50+

physical activity to control BP. This differs from the recommendations for improving aerobic capacity, which involve more intense aerobics activity (80–85% MHR). At higher intensities, BP in HTN (hypertension) people does not decrease.

All Types of Exercise

Whatever the choice of exercise you select, it is important to follow some basic guidelines, not only to maximize your overall health potential but also to avoid exacerbating or even creating health problems.

The Golden Rules of Exercise

The following rules for exercise are mostly a matter of common sense but are very important, nevertheless, and should not be overlooked in any haste to achieve improved levels of fitness.

Rule I: Keep in mind the importance of good equipment and hydration

Do not allow the system to overheat. As someone on a regular exercise program, you will need the cooling effects of fresh water: for each hour of exercise you should drink one half liter of fresh water and a cup of orange juice (for the potassium), 30 minutes *before* beginning the exercise. Dehydration, whether deliberate (by wearing rubberized clothing or excessive use of saunas) or accidental, is not recommended. The resultant weight loss is temporary and will be regained through proper rehydration. Salt tablets are not necessary.

Rule 2 : Prepare your body properly for exertion

Warming up the muscles improves circulation by decreasing the viscosity (thickness) of the blood, making it flow more smoothly through arteries and veins. A proper warm-up and cool-down is important for two reasons. First, it can improve performance by up to 10% by decreasing muscle stiffness and soreness. Second, and more importantly, it helps to avoid irregular heartbeats that abrupt physical exercise can precipitate. The best warm-up is a slow-motion version of the activity you will be practicing. For example, if you are a runner, walk briskly for 3–5 minutes and then break into a jog, then run.

The same is true of cooling down after exercise. Five minutes of warm-up and cool-down is sufficient, and in either case brisk walking is ideal, as it prevents the "pooling" of blood in the legs. Proper cooling down allows circulation to recovering muscles to help clear metabolic waste products like lactic acid.

Rule 3 : Find people you like to exercise with and set realistic goals

There are many forms of exercise to choose from; you should find an activity you enjoy enough to participate in regularly.

Rule 4 : If pain (any type) starts, you STOP!

Again, pay attention to the signal coming from the body so as to avoid fatal accidents. Pain is Nature's way of telling you to slow down.

Rule 5 : Regularity is the key

Being a strictly "weekend athlete" only invites accidents that will discourage a real chance of achieving lasting cardiovascular conditioning.

Rule 6 : Watch heatstroke

The combination of severe heat, humidity and exercise can result in markedly compromised performance and even illness if not properly prepared for: never underestimate the devastating potential of this combination. Follow these guidelines:

■ **Preparation**: if at all possible, exercise in the cooler hours of early morning or in the evening. Not only will the heat be less oppressive, but the amount of carbon monoxide and ozone will be less because most cars will be off the road.

> *Being a strictly "weekend athlete" only invites accidents that will discourage a real chance of achieving lasting cardiovascular conditioning*

- **Hydration**: in severe circumstances, we can sweat up to 2 liters/hour of exercise. That's a significant loss. Just weigh yourself before and after a run or jog and see the difference: that's all water loss! Solution: drink as much as possible 30 minutes prior to exercise (don't worry, water empties from the stomach instantaneously). Then, throughout the exercise, drink 30 ml (a large glass) of fresh water every 30 minutes. Tip: monitor the spittle production – it should be clear, not white.
- **Clothing**: wear loose-fitting cotton clothing that is light colored (reflects the heat better).

Rule 7: Watch athlete's foot and crotch

Fungal infections are very common among athletes, especially in areas of the body where it is moist, dark and warm. Your feet and groin area are perfect for fungal overgrowth, especially if the area involved is kept warm, dark and moist by wearing clothing that does not "breathe."
In general:

- decrease exposure to the locker room fungal colony: wear rubber sandals in the shower;
- clothing: cotton, cotton, cotton! Always wear underwear and socks;
- try topical cream or talc: if itching or redness persists, consult your generalist or podiatrist;
- keep the affected area dry, particularly after a shower;
- try a vinegar soak on the feet: 1 part vinegar and 10 parts water twice a day to dry the area.

Rule 8: Determine, with your doctor's assistance, if regular exercise is safe for you

Although these conditions are relatively uncommon in the general population, there are some physical conditions for which *intense exercise is contra-indicated* (see Table 4.4).

Jumping Rope

It was not until I had been traveling around the globe giving seminars and booking in and out of glass and marble hotels that I started to get tired of fitness centers. They are fine for the occasional sauna or weight training session, but I yearned for a more spontaneous individual workout. Then, an executive

TABLE 4.4 *Conditions for which intense exercise is contra-indicated*

Heart problems

Malignant or accelerated hypertension
Unstable angina or acute heart attack
Unstable heart failure or valvular problems
Unstable rhythms
Aortic aneurysm or dissection

Lung problems

Embolism
Unstable asthma
Pulmonary hypertension

Other

Unstable pregnancy
Unstable diabetes or thyroid disease

at INSEAD, while on a course, lent me his jump rope. I had done it with my sisters as a child but not since and was surprised how a marathon runner could lack the necessary skills to skip rope. Once I tried, I was hooked.

At first, I could do only a minute or so at a rate of 60 skips/minute. Now, I carry the rope with me on my travels and it makes for a very fun workout as I seek out little parks in the cities I am visiting where I can improve my jumping skills.

Equipment

First, watch a video of Sugar Ray Leonard or any top boxer. Get a leather rope or one from a coated wire cable (for speed) of 2.85 meters in length. Check the handles have ball bearings to make the swing smooth. For footwear, I prefer very light old running shoes. At the beginning, you may need long jogging pants as the leather rope may inadvertently slap your leg, causing a distraction.

Training technique

Start slowly, not just to avoid accidents, but to give yourself a chance to develop the patience and skills necessary to have fun while setting back the biological clock. First, stretch a bit, left and right laterally and forward. Do not take an extra step when jumping the rope. Aim for the following progression:

- **First two weeks**: satisfy yourself with getting up to 2 minutes at about 60 jumps/minute. Most people cannot jump for more than 2 minutes continuously without having to stop and catch their breath. Your feet should only come 1 inch off the ground – it is supposed to be a low-impact exercise.

- **Second two weeks**: satisfy yourself with getting up to 4 minutes at about 60 jumps/minute.

- **After one month**: bring your jump rope with you traveling, to bring out in parks and health clubs. Start doing longer and longer times, while mixing in crossovers (like boxers do).

Real benefits of jumping rope

As well as being fun, jumping rope provides some real health benefits:

- it is affordable, portable, safe, fun and effective for everybody;
- it helps to prevent osteoporosis and heart disease;
- it is a total body workout, working the upper and lower body simultaneously;
- it improves your overall strength and stamina levels;
- it helps to improve overall body coordination, agility, balance, and hand–eye coordination as well.

Strength Training

Research has shown that strength training has the following principal benefits:

As you age, your fat compartment grows and your lean compartment (muscles and bones) shrinks

- **Improves your metabolic rate**: this is vitally important for body fat control (see Chapter 1). As you age, your fat compartment grows and your lean compartment (muscles and bones) shrinks. Muscle mass, a part of your lean mass compartment, is a very active tissue, burning up to 100 calories per kilogram *daily*! Therefore, increases in the muscle mass compartment = increases in metabolic rate.

- **Increases your energy and stamina**: a better conditioned musculoskeletal system enables you to go about your daily chores without nagging episodes of fatigue.

- **Improves overall musculoskeletal coordination and balance**: weight training in the older groups improves walking velocity, balance, strength and stamina.
- **Increases the mass of bones**: this helps to ward off osteoporosis, a major cause of illness in older age groups.
- **Improves self-image**: and, possibly, self-confidence.

Provisos

Several provisos are in order with regard to muscular endurance training:

- In terms of sequencing, always perform muscular training exercises after any aerobic sessions because such exercises prior to an aerobic session create an oxygen debt (causing premature fatigue).
- The American College of Sports Medicine warns that strength (weight) training can raise blood pressure, put pressure on the heart, and overall oxygen requirements. Heavy lifts can cause fainting (due to decreased venous return and decreased blood flow to the heart and brain). Exhalation on effort should be encouraged.

When to train

Strength training should always come after aerobic exercise, such as jogging. This is because strength training can help you to incur an oxygen debt, leading to fatigue later on.

How to train

To minimize injuries and improve overall performance, every muscle group should be exercised. There are two major muscle groups to be exercised on alternate days:

- **Upper body**: chest, abdominals, arms (biceps and triceps), shoulders and back.
- **Lower body**: abdominals, thighs, buttocks and calves.

Technical terms

The following terms are commonly used in relation to strength training:

- **Reps (repetitions)**: the number of times that the exercise is to be performed sequentially; for example, doing 10 reps of biceps curls means doing that exercise 10 times without stopping.

- **Sets**: groups of reps; for example, doing three sets of 15 reps of biceps curls means doing the above exercise three times with a break between.

Objectives

The purpose of strength training is to increase:

- **Strength**: accomplished by doing many reps with lighter weights.
- **Mass**: accomplished by doing many reps with heavier weights.

Use either free weights (barbell or dumbbells) or resistance machines, according to your liking.

Getting ready

There are some basic preparations you can undertake before embarking on strength training:

- **Hydration and warm-up**: as for FIT, plus some loose stretching to limber up.
- **Nutrition**: shift the bulk of daily calories from carbohydrates to proteins for muscle reparation.

General movements

The following tips are worth remembering:

- Rest 45–60 seconds between sets: stretch the muscles between sets.
- Instead of using rhythm or momentum to move the weight, be deliberate and take about 2–3 seconds for a complete movement, such as a squat or curl. You should feel the muscle fibers pulling gently, almost burning.
- At the "top" of each movement, squeeze the muscle (contract it hard) for extra mass.

Progression

To benefit fully from strength training, the resistance (weights) must regularly be increased as the muscles quickly adapt to the lower weights.

A good rule of thumb is to start with two sets at the beginning. When the recommended reps are easily achieved, add an extra set, for a maximal number of three sets. Then when that routine becomes easy to do, add

TABLE 4.5 *Alternate-day strength training*

Upper body	Reps	Sets	Weight (men/ women)
1 Chest:			
Lateral wings (see below)	12–15	3	5 kg/3kg
Bench press	12–15	2	30 kg/20 kg
2 Biceps:			
Preacher's curl (see below)	12–15	3	5 kg/3 kg
3 Triceps:			
Press-ups (see p. 107)	your age or >	3	–
Chair dips (see p. 108)	your age or >	3	–
4 Shoulders: Lateral elevations (see below)	10	3	5 kg/3 kg
Chin-ups	Maximum (5+)	3	–

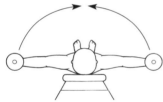

Lateral wings

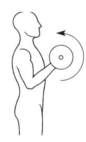

Preacher's curl

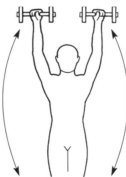

Lateral elevations

5% weight. Once again, when the muscles get used to this new load (within a month or two), add 5% more weight and continue until you have achieved the strength (gauged by the weight you can lift) or mass (gauged by measuring circumferences).

Having a Healthy Pain-Free Back

The common folklore is that bad backs are reserved for those who make a living moving pianos. According to the medical journal *Spine,* more than 80% of people in industrialized countries will be debilitated by this problem some time in their adult lives. In fact, the more sedentary you are, the greater your risk of developing severe back problems. That makes most of us at high risk to develop back pain that will limit our mobility, both on the tennis court and in our jobs.

The more sedentary you are, the greater your risk for developing severe back problems

Moreover, back pain means a major loss of money to companies due to days off work. In the USA alone, back ailments, as the second leading reason for hospitalization (after pregnancy), cost industry *$14 billion per year*, including 93 million lost working days.

What Causes Back Pain

A brief review of the back anatomy reveals both problems and solutions.

The vertebral bodies are the bony building blocks, 33 in all, stacked and interlocked one atop another. Between these vertebrae are rubbery fluid-filled discs, which cushion the weight of the upper body. Then there are muscles (roughly 140) and ligaments, like the stays of a sailboat mast, which hold the spine erect in a natural flattened S-curve, the optimal configuration for flexibility, weight bearing and shock absorption. In the upright position, the spinal cord and the sensitive nerves run just behind these discs in such a way as to be pinched by the compressed disc pushing backwards when you bend forward.

As long as the concave curve in the lower back is preserved, the disc, in most circumstances, tolerates the compression that comes from the pressure of the body's weight. Problems begin when you eliminate that inward curve of the lower back by habitually bending forward, thus compressing, and possibly herniating, the disc backwards.

To complicate matters further, enter the major technological advances of this century: the TV, telephone, computer and automobile and you have the worse activity possible for the back – *long-term sitting*. Though you may be committed to a livelihood that requires you to spend a lot of time on your backside, you need not be one of the 80% of back sufferers cited above. Table 4.6 gives some of the common causes of back pain.

TABLE 4.6 *Some of the common causes of back pain*

Problem	Cause (s)	Comments
Slipped (herniated) disc/muscle strain	1 Accidents or trauma 2 Poor posture/bending 3 Obesity 4 Poor abdominal tone 5 Twisting while lifting 6 Falling	1 Learn to lift and bend well: bend knees! 2 Improve abdominal muscle tone 3 Consider yoga
Osteoporosis	Demineralization of vertebral bodies in back due to: a) Excess calcium loss due to excess use of diuretics like caffeine and alcohol b) Decreased intake of calcium or Vitamin D	1 Maintain bone mass through exercises such as walking or weight training and by adequate calcium intake 2 Decrease caffeine and alcohol intake 3 Get plenty of sunshine
Degenerative joint disease	Simple wear and tear: repeated trauma due to sports injuries or child bearing	Maintain back suppleness by performing yoga or stretching exercises
Ankylosing spondylitis	Heredity	

Before Developing Acute Back Pain …

The following are some key guidelines to remaining free from this scourge of the 21st century:

1 *Watch the posture*: by maintaining the natural S-shaped curve to the back, you not only keep the muscles strong, but you stay mentally focussed. That is, your posture will determine in large part your attitude and inner chemistry by sending internal signals that you are either in control (shoulders back, head high) or dejected and beaten (stooped shoulders, head down).

2 *Regular aerobic exercise*: crucial to maintain the strength of the back muscles. Brisk walking is ideal. Complement these activities with some night-time stretching or yoga.

3 *Get rid of that potbelly*: get the body fat under control. Added fat distributed up-front will only put more strain on the back muscles. Moreover, the spine receives most of its mechanical support from the massive abdominal musculature, not the back muscles themselves. Tone up the abdominal muscles by flexing them while sitting on planes, lifting and driving.

While driving on long hauls, keep the knees higher than the pelvis. Maintain the natural curve of your spine by placing a cushion or a rolled-up towel behind your lower back to lend support. Do not twist when getting in and out of your car. When driving, realign the back every hour or so by standing, with hands placed on the lower back, and bending backwards.

4 *Lift objects properly*: perform the "marble test." In the morning of a normal work day, put a smart marble in your breast pocket. During the day, if the marble rolls out of your pocket, that is because you bent over *at the waist*, instead of squatting to pick something up. Above all, do not bend over to pick something or someone up: let your legs do the bending. When lifting, keep the object very close to your body. Lift twice: once in your mind, visualizing the best way to do it, and then in reality. This will help to avoid the reflex of bending over to pick something up.

Moreover, bending your legs will build powerful leg muscles and this is important to your heart. When the heart pumps blood to the lower body and legs, it does so with the help of gravity. Getting the blood back to the lungs requires more assistance as the blood flow is now going against gravity. Strong leg muscles can help by "milking" the blood in the veins upwards. Strong legs, therefore, can act not only to save the back but also as a second heart!

5 *While sitting in your car or at your desk*: sit up and avoid stooping. The natural contour of the back is that of an "S," not an "I" (too straight) and definitely not a "C" (stooping crushes the internal organs). During the day, tense your abdominal muscles to give them the strength they need to support your back. Be certain that your chair supports your lower back well.

6 *While travelling*: divide the weight of your bags evenly so as to not strain one side more than the other. Likewise, instead of carrying a mammoth single bag, consider carrying two lighter bags.

7 *Sleep the right way*: find the ideal situation for the back. Sleep on your side with the top leg bent and bottom leg straight, using a firm mattress or tatami.

8 *Women beware*: high heels throw the back into an exaggerated position. Thought by some to be sexy, they should come with traction devices.

9 *Best single exercise for preventing back pain*: the abdominal "crunch" (see p. 105). So called, because you only lift your shoulder blades off the floor about 10–15° – no more! This action selectively strengthens the rectus abdominus muscles (those abdominal muscles in front known by body builders as the "six-pack") and provides frontal support to the lower back. Do this slowly and completely until you feel the muscle "burn" and then do five more. As a variant to the above maneuver, tilt to the left and right side while coming up. This will strengthen the internal and external oblique muscle groups that act as a girdle to the side aspect of the abdomen.

Once You Develop Acute Back Pain …

If you have already developed acute back pain, you will want to seek relief both immediately and for the longer term.

Back pain relief in seconds

If the back pain is more like a nagging stiffness that prevents a full range of motion, try this to stave off the final back crisis (this maneuver is called the "Indian squat"): Standing normally with the feet slightly separated, arms raised in front of you, begin to bend the knees to come down to the squatting position shown on page 130. Gently squat as far down as you can, while keeping your heels flat on the floor. While feeling the stretching in the lower back, push against the inner thighs with the elbows. Hold that position for 15 seconds. Repeat as necessary.

If you cannot squat this way, hold on to something strong and feel the muscles stretching.

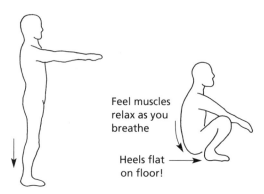

Feel muscles
relax as you
breathe

Heels flat ⟶
on floor!

Important health note: to be effective in smoothing out the back muscles, the heels *must* be kept on the floor. You may keep the arms extended out in front of you and even, in the early stages of building flexibility, stabilize yourself by holding on to the bathtub or a tree trunk. Eventually, however, you will want, once you get into the full squatting position with heels on the floor, to tuck your elbows in between the thighs and stretch the thigh muscles outwards. Back stiffness will subside after several seconds in this position and, if followed by a warm bath with Epsom salts and repeated before bedtime, a possible back crisis will have been averted.

Alternatively, there is a whole array of therapeutic modalities (massage, hot water bottle, manipulation, acupuncture, ultrasound deep heat, traction, shoe inserts, surgery), none of which are 100% successful. In fact, most back pain subsides, regardless of any approach such as bedrest, aspirin and the tincture of time. Otherwise, see your doctor for further investigation, particularly if pain is accompanied by fever. With a little care and forethought, you will defy the adage: "Once a back patient, always a back patient."

Back flexibility plan

Think about aging for a moment. One of the images that arises will be of stiffness, neck stiffness (Grandpa backing out of the driveway!), back stiffness, artery stiffness and attitude stiffness. Remember: *never bounce* when you stretch. It leads to small tears in your muscles. Just feel a gentle pull and maintain that position for 30 seconds. The duration is much more important than the intensity of the stretch. Gain extra benefits by following your breaths, in and out, for the entire 30 second count. Concentrate on them instead of on the muscles.

This evening, while preparing for bed, look into the dressing mirrror and say with conviction: "Meet the new Mr (or Mrs) Elastic, supple and lithe, able to play sports such as football with the kids, vibrant sex partner, nimble of body and mind!" It's yours in four weeks by following this regimen:

1 *Lateral stretch* (see p. 104):15 seconds right and 15 seconds left side, while breathing deeply and smiling. Staying in one plane, without leaning forward or back, legs spread as wide as comfortable, slide your lead arm down leg until you feel a slight sticking resistance from the muscles and tendons.

> Later in life, you may not want to run a marathon, but you will want to bend over and tie your shoe or hold your grandchild. Yoga is the prime example of this type of training.

2 *Knee-to-chest chest*: bring your thigh as close to your chest as you can. Hold it for a count of 10. Repeat with other leg. Breathe! Now, bring both thighs as close to your chest as you can. Hold for a count of 10. Breathe through.

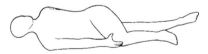

One knee to chest

Both knees to chest

3 *Stretch for lower back and hip*: keep your hips and shoulders on the floor and gently press down with your hand on your bent knee toward the floor. Hold for a count of 15. Repeat with other leg.

4 *Sit with your right leg straight*: bend your left leg and cross your left foot over your outstretched right leg. Then bend your right elbow and rest it on the outside of your left knee. Now with your left hand straightened behind you, slowly turn your head to look over your left shoulder and rotate your upper body in the same direction. To get a better stretch as you rotate your upper body to the left, gently push your left knee with

your elbow to the right. Hold that position for 15 seconds. Repeat with other side. Do not ever hold your breath–breathe through.

5 *Half-cobra (spine stretch)*: lie face down on the floor and completely relax the spine. Raise up your head first, then raise the top part of your torso off the floor, using only the back muscles for lift. Keep the lower part of your abdomen on the floor and relax the neck and shoulder muscles. Keep breathing and smiling. Hold the cobra position for a count of 20 seconds.

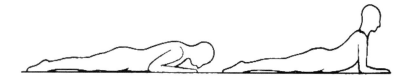

6 *Salute to the sun*: a more advanced group of movements linked to integrate mind and body health nicely in just a few minutes.

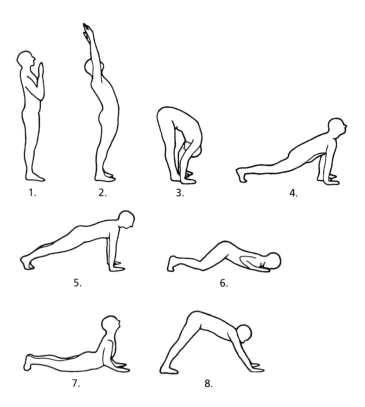

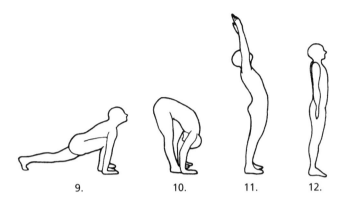

9.   10.   11.   12.

Immediate Things to Do/Buy to Get Going Right Now!

Get up off of that thing. Then you'll feel better!

JAMES BROWN

- Attitude-wise: do not allow anyone to convince you, do it for yourself.
- Have a teenage son? Immediately buy (a) two pairs of boxing gloves and (b) a pair of ballet slippers, and allow him to choose.
- Buy a *leather* jump rope, with screw-in weights for handles.
- Hang a horizontal chin-up bar in your office and home. You are not wasting your money, it *will* get used.
- Free weight set: 2, 5, 10 kg (with simple bench and (optional) rock music.
- Until you have figured a way around hundreds of e-mails daily, while e-mailing, get up and do the lateral stretches described on page 104.

TIPS FOR YOUR HEALTH ACTION PLAN

The best time to work out ... early morning: high resolve and motivation, high oxygen

The best way to get in shape in only 30 seconds . .. a chin-up bar (also the cheapest)

The best way to improve abdominal tone ... the crunch + abdominal snap

The best hotel workout ... yoga, skipping rope, 4-minute workout

The best maneuver for back stiffness ... the Indian squat
The best maneuver for back pain ... the knees-to-chest maneuver
The best exercise for preventing back pain ... the abdominal crunch:
   (curl-ups)

Frequently Asked Questions

Exercise (General)

Q What is the **minimum** necessary?

■ Before you even buy a pair of running shoes or leotard, read Chapter 6 to avoid getting into the messy world of guilt. According to recent research,[2] for those men walking briskly only three or more times per week there was a 10% reduction in risk of heart disease. Walk briskly after meals six times a week and experience a linear risk reduction.

Q What indoor exercise **equipment** should I buy?

■ Consider investing in the following equipment, particularly if you live where the weather is cold and wet, have a family and a little space:
   - **Treadmill**: get one with a real motor (1–2 horsepower is best) as walking briskly up an incline of 10–20° is comparable to jogging. *Comment*: make sure that the handrails can support you while you are running.
   - **Rowers**: these exercise not just the upper body; in fact, if properly done, the work done by the extension of the leg can be up to 75% of the total work done. *Comment*: try the wind-resistance type (more natural) and watch the back by pulling the elbows tight against the body during the pulling phase.
   - **Stationary bicycle**: try the ones with a friction belt or wind as resistance. *Comment*: (a) the seated models are easier on the back; (b) use the pedal rat traps to exercise both the muscles in the front and the back of the leg; and (c) adjust the seat so that your knee is slightly bent (160°) to prevent undue wear on the knee.
   - **Stair-climbers**: expensive choice. *Comment*: keep your knees over the feet, the back straight and the arms lightly on the handrails for the optimal workout.
   - **Ski simulators**: the most intense workout, using both the upper and lower body. *Comment*: considerable skill is required, and for non-skiers this may be an obstacle.

Q When should I do a workout?

■ Any time during the day that suits you. If you cannot work out, eat light and walk.

Q Is **4 minutes** long enough to condition the body?

■ Done properly, our research indicates that the 4-minute workout prepares both the body and the mind for the inherent stresses facing the business community.

Q Why can't I **sleep** well after activity?

■ You are overexcited. Do the workout in the morning.

Q How safe are **health clubs**?

■ In a series of random surveys of fitness clubs in the USA, researchers found that many (28%) failed to screen new members to identify potential risks, 92% failed to conduct emergency drills, and 60% had no written medical emergency-response plans available. Recommendations by the American Heart Association include the above measures, together with full certification in cardio-pulmonary resuscitation (CPR). Gyms could invest in defibrillators[3] as well, since their populations are getting older and older.

Q Am I actually increasing the **quantity** of my life by being health conscious?

■ You are improving not just the quantity but the quality as well. Researchers studied the medical records of 366,000 people in Chicago to determine the effects of pursuing a "low-risk lifestyle" (BP at 120/80 or lower, no cigarettes, total cholesterol < 2.0 grams/liter, and no diabetes or known heart disease).[4] Their health was tracked for 20 years during which 38,000 died. The conclusion:
  – low-risk men under 40: 89% lower death rate from coronary artery disease over others in age group; *no* deaths from stroke;
  – low-risk men aged 40–59: 64% less strokes than higher-risk men;
  – overall low-risk men had a 50% lower death rate from cancer, low-risk women had a 17% lower death rate from cancer;
  – low-risk men and women aged 40–59: 78% lower death rate.

Exercise: Sex

Q Does sex count as **exercise**?

■ Sex can help to condition the heart as long as it follows the FIT prescription described within this chapter:
  - Frequency: two to three times per week;
  - Intensity: at your training heart rate;
  - Time: for (at least) 20 minutes.

Q Is sex safe after a **heart attack**?

■ Yes, in fact, love-making should be prescribed for patients with a heart problem in the same way that we prescribe pure nutrition, medications and exercise. In a study of more than 850 men and women who had survived heart attacks, it was demonstrated the chance of provoking a heart attack with sex was less than 2/1,000,000! This is particularly true if sex is supplemented with a regular walking program, as the well-conditioned muscular system is more efficient in extracting oxygen from the blood and delivering it to the heart.

Stamina and Fatigue

Q What are the most **time-efficient** ways to gain real stamina?

■ There are three key ingredients to achieving high stamina – attitude, exercise and nutrition:
  - Work not from compulsion (that's workaholism), but from the enthusiasm that comes with being part of the dynamic world economy. Staying excited about life will keep your energy focussed.
  - Avoid confused and cynical people: it will demoralize and de-energize you.
  - Surround yourself with people with a sense of mission and grand design: the fastest way to get energized.
  - As the day wears on and you notice your first yawn, take five deep breaths, 45 (or your age) desk press-ups or curl-ups and five deep breaths again. Alternatively, catch a cat nap (drop your head to your chest, smile and let go in the taxi on the way to the airport or while waiting).
  - Drink: lots of water and freshly squeezed juice. Replace coffee with kiwi juice with Vitamin C crystals. Avoid carbohydrates because they tend to raise blood levels of serotonin, a natural tranquilizer for the brain.

Q Am I **exercising too much**?

■ Not if you are free of these cardinal signs of overtraining:
 – body fat < 5%;
 – soreness, injuries, frequent infections, high pulse (> 68 beats/minute);
 – moodiness, depression, fatigue, insomnia, low appetite.

Q My friend said we all should do some **jogging**, but I cannot stand it. Ideas?

■ To determine the physical exercise most appropriate for you, do an exercise. Imagine your genetic ancestors, many thousands of years ago, sitting around a camp fire. We are all descendants from various tribal forebears and, as such, we all had roles: some of our forebears were group hunters, some were lone hunters, some were gatherers, some were planners, and some of them were care givers. Everybody had a role that best suited their personality and body habits. Running is for the ancestral hunters while walking is for everyone, at all ages, regardless of health status.

Q I could use some challenging, yet feasible, fitness **goals**. Ideas?

■ For the **novice**:
 – run 3 miles in under 30 minutes;
 – cycle 20 miles in 90 minutes;
 – hike 12 miles in 3 hours;
 – bench-press your weight;
 – chin-ups 25/ day.

■ For the **intermediate** player:
 – hike on weekends;
 – ride a century (100 km);
 – chin-ups 10/ minute or 35/day;
 – run a marathon[3] under $3\frac{1}{2}$ hours.

■ For the **advanced** athlete:
 – play football league;
 – climb a mountain.

SELF-ASSESSMENT QUIZ

1 The best time to exercise:

(a) am

(b) pm

Hint: Motivation is higher

2 If I exercise in the afternoon, there is no need to walk after dinner:

(a) True

(b) False

Hint: Metabolic rate stays elevated for a long while after the workout

3 To practice yoga correctly, one must be religious:

(a) True

(b) False

Hint: Body flexibility = mind flexibility

4 You are Stage I (beginner) if:

(a) BP > 160/100

(b) TG:HDL > 5

(c) You smoke 20 cigarettes or more a day

(d) LDL > 1.60 g/l

(e) BF > 25%

(f) CF > 130 beats

5 You are Stage II (intermediate) if:

(a) BP < 140/90

(b) TG:HDL > 3 –5

(c) You smoke 10–20 cigarettes a day

(d) LDL 1.30–1.60 g/l

(e) BF 20–25%

6 You are Stage III (advanced) if:

(a) BP < 135/85

(b) TG:HDL < 3

(c) You don't smoke

(d) LDL < 1.30 g/L

(e) BF < 20%

(f) CF < 100 beats

7 Between the ages of 20 years and 60 years, we lose on average _____ % of our heart efficiency (fitness):

(a) 10%
(b) 20%
(c) 30%
(d) 40%

Hint: If you don't use it, you lose it!

8 Aging markers:

(a) Lack of flexibility
(b) Hair loss
(c) Gray hair
(d) Wrinkles
(e) Skin tone
(f) Attitude

Hint: Everything is expressed in attitude

9 While exercising, you should drink water:

(a) Before the exercise
(b) During the exercise
(c) After the exercise

Hint: Dehydration = fatigue

10 The best foods to eat after a 30-minute workout include:

(a) Spaghetti
(b) Rice
(c) Potatoes
(d) Salads
(e) Green vegetables

Hint: Complete carbohydrates are necessary to restore the balance

Answers

1 (a)   **6** All
2 (a)   **7** (d)
3 (b)   **8** All
4 (a) (d) & (f)   **9** All
5 (b) (c) (d) & (e)   **10** (a) (b) (c) & (e)

Notes

1   Optimal sexuality is as good as any motivator (and better than most). Although sexual expression is obviously a complex and highly individualized affair, essentially what is happening is that we are using the body to connect with our partners, to lose our separation: an emotional and physical meltdown. It helps to have a body that can manage its way through physical intimacy. So, exercise can increase your endurance and optimize your body fat so that a pleasurable experience lasts even longer and is more intense. That's because of the effect of regular aerobic exercise on the reproductive and cardiovascular systems: muscles are better toned and conditioned, arteries supplying the sexual organs are open and delivering oxygen and glucose to the penis better, and men have higher testosterone in the blood. All these effects are important in maintaining erections. Psychologically, a toned body also provides the necessary confidence and self-esteem to allow you to let the body "do its thing" without a lot of neurotic interference.

2   Harvard Alumni Study, *Circulation*, 2000, Aug.

3   Defibrillators (now fully automated) help the heart regain its normal rhythm after a heart attack, but must be used by competent individuals because the chances of survival decrease 7–10% for every minute lost before defibrillation.

4   *Journal of the American Medical Association*, 1999, Dec.

5   Marathon: a Greek village 24 miles from Athens and the site of a decisive battle in 490 BC between the grossly outnumbered Greek warriors and the Persian forces of Darius the Great. Legend has it that the Greek commanders instructed the runner Pheidippides to run 150 miles to Sparta to get reinforcements. Then, they instructed him to run the additional 24 miles across the Plains of Marathon to inform the Athenians of the victory, whereupon he collapsed and died. The distance was extended in the 1908 Olympic Games in London to 26 miles 385 yards, so that the royal family could encourage the runners from their royal box.

CHAPTER FIVE

WORRYING EFFECTIVELY

▶▶▶▶▶ ▶▶▶▶▶▶▶▶▶▶▶▶ ▶ ▶▶▶▶▶▶▶▶▶▶▶▶▶▶ ▶

The paradox of our time in history is that we have taller buildings, but shorter tempers; wider freeways, but narrower viewpoints. We spend more, but have less; we buy more, but enjoy it less. We have bigger houses and smaller families; more conveniences, but less time; we have more degrees, but less sense; more knowledge, but less judgement; more experts, but more problems; more medicine, but less wellness. We drink too much, smoke too much, spend too recklessly, laugh too little, drive too fast, get too angry too quickly, stay up too late, get up too tired, read too seldom, watch TV too much, and pray too seldom. We have multiplied our possessions, but reduced our values. We talk too much, love too seldom, and hate too often. We've learned how to make a living, but not a life; we've added years to life, not life to years. We've been all the way to the moon and back, but have trouble crossing the street to meet the new neighbor. We've conquered outer space, but not inner space. We've done larger things, but not better things. We've cleaned up the air, but polluted the soul. We've split the atom, but not our prejudice. We write more, but learn less. We plan more, but accomplish less. We've learned to rush, but not to wait. We build more computers to hold more information to produce more copies than ever, but have less communication. These are the times of fast foods and slow digestion; tall men and short character; steep profits and shallow relationships. These are the times of world peace, but domestic warfare; more leisure, but less fun; more kinds of food, but less nutrition. These are days of two incomes, but more divorce; of fancier houses, but broken homes. These are days of quick trips, disposable diapers, throw-away morality, one-night stands, overweight bodies, and pills that do everything from cheer to quiet, to kill.

GEORGE CARLIN

Using the advice contained in this chapter, Mr Timebomb could take care of the following health issues :

- prevent stress from permanently damaging health
- body fat
- high cholesterol
- high blood triglycerides
- low HDL (good) cholesterol
- low stamina
- regain the smile on his face, decrease his furrowed brow.

What is Worrying Us ?

Today's business environment (hostile takeovers, acquisitions, mergers, deregulation, downsizing uncertainty and the new technologies) can produce changes in our lives with more speed and violence than ever before. Who will survive? Who will thrive? Aspects of our life that once provided shelter and refuge (job security, our health, marriages and other relationships) are all now vulnerable. This chapter addresses not just the classic external sources of stress, but also presents tried and true strategies for surviving our own internal neuroses.

As part of our ongoing research at INSEAD on the health implications of stress within corporations, we have asked more than 30,000 managers from all over the world what they consider to be the principal causes of worry in their lives. Across 40 countries and 400 corporations, the responses were remarkably uniform (there was virtually no significant difference among cultures, races, genders). (See Table 5.1.)

Health and the Changes of Life

In order to measure the relationship between the magnitude of life changes and health, Holmes and Rahe[1] used a schedule of recent experience. This is called the Life Event Survey, which can help to correlate the accumulated risk and impact of life changes on health and disease. Using this survey (shown in Table 5.2) indicate which, if any, of the following stresses of life you have experienced *within the last 12 months* and then calculate your score.

TABLE 5.1 *The classic worries of 30,000 managers (1989–2001)*

Family issues	%
Health and safety of loved ones	93
Children's choice of friends, school performance/overall values	76
Partner issues: marital discord	56

Self	%
Achieving career ambitions	68
Self-imposed pressures: money (getting it, saving it), time pressures, traffic	63
Death	54
Aging	51
Self-doubt	52
Lack of personal flexibility	52
Isolation	32

Work issues	%
Fear of failure at work	65
Unrealistic deadlines	60
Excessive demands (excess e-mails/phone calls/meetings)	45
Being made redundant	45
Role conflicts/unreasonable people	39
Absence of support	35
Job incompatibility	34
Compensation issues	13

The research by Holmes and Rahe showed that for those whose changes came too fast or too severe, such as that group who scored more than 300, the chance of developing a minor illness in the near future (within a three-month period) was about 80%; 50% in those who scored between 150 and 299 and 30% in those who scored less than 150. The severity of the illness corresponded to the score. These diseases ranged from serious diseases like heart diseases, ulcer disease, diabetes, alcoholism, cancers, depression, suicide and certain infections, to less life-threatening annoyances, such as the common cold and indigestion.

Another lesson to be picked up here is that, despite all the neurotic worrying we do about these changes, the vast majority of us are very lucky indeed. So often do we extrapolate small complaints or symptoms into the full-blown disease. The loved one is dead and buried ten times over before the doctor is even called! We invite sleepless nights by not simply counting our blessings and taking one day at a time.

TABLE 5.2 *Social readjustments rating scale (Holmes and Rahe)*

Event	Rating
Death of a spouse	100
Divorce	73
Marital separation	65
Jail term	63
Death of a close family member	63
Personal illness or injury	53
Getting married	50
Fired at work	47
Marital reconciliation	45
Retirement	45
Change in health of family member	44
Pregnancy	40
Sexual difficulties	39
Gaining a new family member	39
Business readjustment	39
Change in financial status	38
Death of close friend	37
Change in type of work	36
Arguments with spouse	35
High mortgage	31
Foreclosure of a loan	30
Change in responsibilities at work	29
Child leaving home	29
Trouble with in-laws	29
Outstanding personal achievement	28
Spouse begins or stops work	28
Beginning or ending education	26
Change in living conditions	25
Change in personal habits	24
Trouble with boss	23
Change in work conditions	20
Expatriation/repatriation	20
Change in place of education	20
Change in recreation	19
Change in church activities	19
Change in social activities	18
Change in sleeping habits	16
Change in number of family meetings	15
Change in eating habits	15
Vacation	13
Minor violations of the law	11
Total up your LES score here	**Total:** ____

Is Being Type A Really Worth It?

Early in the 1960s a large body of retrospective and prospective evidence began accumulating in support of an independent impact of the Type A Behavior Pattern (TABP)[2] on health, particularly the development of heart disease, stroke, and cancers. What are the facts regarding this link between personality (software) and disease ?

To start off, it was discovered that only 60% of all heart attacks are due to the usual risk factors: blood pressure, cigarettes, cholesterol, obesity and low physical activity. The other 40% are due to mental factors such as stress and emotional imbalances. In an effort to understand this personality link to heat disease and strokes, models of personality types were constructed and studied. The strongest components of the TABP associated with heart disease were: hostility,[3] quick anger, irritability, controlling and competitiveness.[4] What are the physiologic results of uncontrolled anger? The scientific studies provide compelling insights:

Only 60% of all heart attacks are due to the usual risk factors; 40% are due to mental factors such as stress and emotional imbalances

1 In a study of 1,600 heart attack victims, researchers found that a previous episode of *anger* within the previous two hours could increase the risk of suffering a heart attack by more than double.

2 A study at Harvard School of Public Health, demonstrated that men (who were free of heart disease at the time of the study) who scored highest on an *anger* scale in a personality profile, had a threefold increase in their risk to develop a heart attack over the subsequent seven years.

3 A study of angioplasty patients revealed that those who scored highest on a *hostility* scale had nearly three times the risk of clogging their newly "cleaned" vessels within a year.

4 Researchers at Arizona State University have proven that people with *smoldering hostility* have greater increases in diastolic blood pressure, a situation that contributes to heart attacks and strokes. The researchers found that people with hostile attitudes have inherent levels of distrust and actually anticipate trouble in relationships – even before there is proof that there is a reason for suspicion.

5 Moreover, a person who is *anger-prone* is about three times more likely to have a heart attack or sudden death than someone with appropriate coping skills.

Type A Behavior Pattern is Not the Only Software in Town

Is your mental software giving you a heart attack? Looking at the person-ality spectra in Table 5.3 and circle the number that best corresponds to your situation. For example, if you are very competitive, you should circle between 7 and 10.

TABLE 5.3 *Assessing your personality type*

Type B											Type A (Coronary-prone)
Not particularly competitive	1	2	3	4	5	6	7	8	9	10	Obsessively competitive, perfectionist[5]
Knows how to wait patiently	1	2	3	4	5	6	7	8	9	10	Upset/insulted by having to wait
Responsive	1	2	3	4	5	6	7	8	9	10	Reactive, irritable, judgemental
Deliberate, even when pressured	1	2	3	4	5	6	7	8	9	10	Always in a hurry, "never late"
Deferential	1	2	3	4	5	6	7	8	9	10	Self-references, emphatic
Well-developed of sense of humor	1	2	3	4	5	6	7	8	9	10	Humorless, serious, rigid
Active listener	1	2	3	4	5	6	7	8	9	10	Tries to finish others' sentences
Takes one thing at a time	1	2	3	4	5	6	7	8	9	10	Polyphasic (five activities at once)
Easygoing, no ambitions	1	2	3	4	5	6	7	8	9	10	Quick tempered, explosive
Present-orientated	1	2	3	4	5	6	7	8	9	10	Past/future-orientated, ambitious
Trust is centerpiece of personality	1	2	3	4	5	6	7	8	9	10	Mistrustful, suspicious

Interpretation: on average, the higher the score, the greater the chance that you have higher adrenaline and cortisol levels, higher blood pressure and heart rate, thicker blood and higher triglycerides. This is why Type A Behavior Pattern (TABP) is also referred to as coronary-prone personality software.

A Heart Attack Begins in the Mind

How does anger translate into heart disease? Our nervous system has not evolved as quickly as our lifestyles. Our bodies cannot tell the difference between mental and physical stress: the same chemical events happen within the body whether you are in *real* or *imagined* danger. As the horse awaits the orders from the rider, the body awaits the orders from the mind. This is where the mind can lead the body by selectively evoking the stress cascade (Figure 5.1).

The primary factor (and the best place to intervene) is the mind, where all disease begins. Paradoxically, this stress cascade is often triggered by those electronic tools that were meant to serve us by helping us use our time more efficiently.

That is, simply by not staying centered and reading an incoming threat from the outside, we provoke the secretion of adrenaline and cortisol by

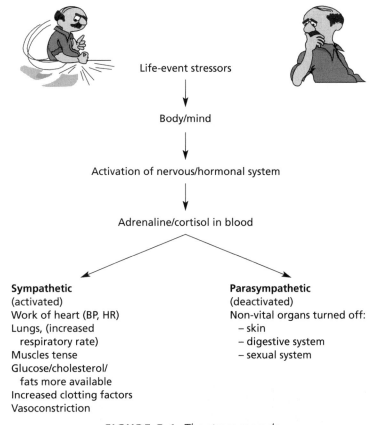

FIGURE 5.1 *The stress cascade*

the adrenal glands, a reaction which was designed originally to enhance the fight-or-flight response and our survival. However, after years of chronic battering of the brain and heart by these stress chemicals, the survival benefits are reversed, with the consequent detrimental effects (see Table 5.4).

TABLE 5.4 *Detrimental effects of adrenaline and cortisol*

Adrenaline effects

Increase of BP: thereby injuring the lining of the coronary/cerebral arteries.
Increase in triglycerides (blood fats).
Increased platelet aggregation (thicker blood).
Increase in artery wall thickness and reactivity.
Lastly, those coronary arteries that have already been stiffened by this arteriosclerosis cannot react to mental stress by dilating and in fact, paradoxically, constrict during mental stress.

Cortisol effects

Increased sensitivity of adrenaline receptors on the heart/ brain.
Increases in production of adrenaline precursors and decreased adrenaline breakdown.
Increased insulin[6] response to sugar.
Dampened and weakened immune function.
Conversion of proteins to fat and carbohydrates (causing insulin surge).
Increased arteriosclerosis.

Make Courage Your Mental Gatekeeper

The novelist Henry James wrote about a man who had a nagging suspicion that something terrible was going to happen to him during his life ... somewhere in his fifties he figured out what that terrible thing was: the terrible thing was that absolutely nothing was going to happen to him. He was going to go through his entire life safely without adventure, without danger, without full participation. And by the time he figured that out, it was too late.

EDWARD ALBEE

The following rules for mustering courage are clear, effective and uncompromising:

1 Accept with enthusiasm any challenge that confronts you. *Never* push trouble away: there are many lessons to be learned and a reputation as an effective troubleshooter is enviable. The most foolish action you could take when confronted by an angry dog is to turn and run. Life is that way, too.

2 Do not yield to the charlatans of self-pity or doubt.[7] They are symptoms of unmanliness. Mastering doubt is part of the offering of life's challenges. Negative feelings in a crisis are merely black clouds, whose transit through our lives can actually be slowed by our fascination with them. Ask yourself: Would you be the person you are today if you had refused even one of life's lessons? Which of your difficult learning experiences would you send back?

3 If you are defeated in this one battle, that should be lesson enough on how to escape the weakness, if escape is indeed the desired end. Face it, all of life up to now has been a series of contrived training sessions for taking risks. You have already done the most courageous thing anyone could do: in being born, you left the maternal ocean to explore this thing called Life. Remove doubt or die a smaller person.

Seeing with New Eyes

Take victimhood, for example. Dump it, as you should have done just after adolescence. The "Why me?" mantra destabilizes positive attitudes.[8] It is a holdover from those days when Mom kept us home from school because we were ill and, while we were recovering, we discovered that being (or playing) weak yields benefits for the victim. Survey your own experience. Do you gain added benefit from playing victim? When life presents a challenging moment, what do you hear inside? (See Table 5.5.)

TABLE 5.5 *Destructive vs constructive mindset*

Destructive (weakened) mindset	Constructive (hardy) mindset
Why me?	Why not? My turn …
Emotional	Disciplined
Cynical, manipulative	Positive, constructive
Reactive	Proactive
Highly stressed and anxious	Highly stressed and serene
Threatened	Assured
Dependent	Self-motivated
Past/future-orientated	Present-orientated: big picture makes sense
Never enough time	Never in a hurry

Absolutely, positively refuse to play victim as a cardinal rule

Absolutely, positively refuse to play victim as a cardinal rule. Slowly and consciously replace one set of thoughts with another and watch things turn around. Within ten days of accepting challenges with enthusiasm, instead of fear, profound and irreversible personal transformation will have started.

Mastering Fear: Hostage No More

Some would argue that fear is the key sign that your faith in the Grand Design is weak and faltering. Faith, simply put, is a re-perception of your *self* (all that you identify with your body and mind within the borders of your skin) as a real part of the Self (the Life Force, Atman, God). Fears, therefore, are just a reminder that perhaps you are not as grand and infinite as you originally thought. As such, fears, if consciously handled, should represent an invitation to strengthen faith, to do internal battle with negative feelings or impulses. Fear could be the starting point of humility over arrogance.

Always keep some aces up your sleeve against fear. One effective fear-buster is the expression: "and so?" Many of our acquired fears stem from a lack of self-confidence in the face of loss: for example, what if I lose my job? With a well-developed sense of adventure, trust in yourself, and the driver, you'll manage just fine. But they'll take my respectability, my spouse, my child, my hair, my youth. It will *all* be stripped away eventually. Newly borns have two innate fears (again, very useful): the fear of falling (being dropped) and the fear of loud noises. The rest we develop as we come up through the stages of life. Fear is the height of arrogance as it presumes that we have to control something that is not ours to control.

Fear is another flawed mindset, left over from adolescence, that presumes that we are the prime mover of everything around us. The US philosopher Ralph Emerson wrote, "Do the thing you are most afraid to do and death of that fear is certain." Though confirmed throughout the ages, it is an experiment that few of us have taken the few minutes to do.

Table 5.6 shows the result of a fear audit that we conducted for several thousand managers between 1997 and 2001. Make your own audit by listing all fears, *imaginary* (including neurotic unfound fear such as going broke or becoming bald) and *real* (falling over a cliff). Now ask yourself: What is worse – fear of baldness or baldness? Strive not to become a lifelong hostage to fear. Start today to fight fears standing up on your feet. When problems arise, spend the first 5 minutes gathering all

TABLE 5.6 *A typical fear audit*

Sources of fear	
Illness of family member	85%
Old age	80%
Death	65%
Work issue	60%
Change	31%
Violence	21%
Unknown	12%

the facts of the matter. Then ask "what's to be done?" or try to get the resolution of the affair under way; then go on to something else. Never worry more than 15 minutes about an affair of money, fame, power, pride or other such earthly trivialities.

John Donne, one of the greatest metaphysical poets, confronts death itself in his sixth *Holy Sonnet*. Memorize this sonnet.

Death be not proud, though some have called thee
Mighty and dreadful, for thou art not so,
For those whom thou think'st thou dost overthrow,
Die not, poor death, nor yet canst thou kill me.
From rest and sleepe, which but thy pictures be,
Much pleasure then from thee, much more must flow,
And soonest our best men with thee do go,
Rest of their bones, and souls' delivery.

Thou'rt slave to Fate, Chance, kings and desperate men,
And dost with poison, war and sickness dwell,
And poppy or charms can make us sleep as well,
And better than thy stroke; why swell'st thou, then?
One short sleep past, we wake eternally,
And death shall be no more: death, thou shalt die.

Watch the Black Dog of Depression

In the USA alone, depression accounts for $129.3 billion in medical care every year, both from lost earnings from lost work time, as well as lost life-time earnings because of depression-induced suicides. A bout of depression will seem all-consuming, all-paralyzing, often lasting up to nine months.

If undiagnosed and untreated, one bout of depression leads to another ever more frequently and severely. However, depression is easily diagnosed and treated. Up to 70% of people suffering from it can be cured by their first attempt at modern treatment. Most of the remaining 30% can be cured by a second or third attempt. There's no reason for anyone to suffer needlessly.

Depression can be diagnosed by establishing that, for most or all of every day for two weeks, a person has experienced at least five of the following ten symptoms:

- emotional instability – sadness with periods of crying;
- feelings of guilt, self-blame;
- changes in sleep pattern (for adults, this usually means falling asleep but waking up earlier than intended, and still tired; for adolescents and young adults, it may mean sleeping much more than usual);
- changes in appetite and weight (adults usually lose; younger patients may eat more and gain);
- decreased interest in sex;
- decreased ability to enjoy things one used to enjoy;
- decreased ability to concentrate;
- decreased energy;
- feelings of hopelessness and helplessness;
- thoughts of death and even suicide.

When nothing else can stop the slide into darkness, take solace in these words from the Hindu sacred text, the *Mundaka Upanishad*:

> *Yea, this is the best of the worlds …*
>
> *Thank the Lord, O moping man, O weeping man, Thank the Lord, O groping man, O thankless man,*

That the world is not different from what it is! Here Karma works: you can do and undo.

Here mettle tells; good is valued. Here austerities bear fruit. Self-application is rewarded.

Sincerity is understood, murder known. Here seeds sprout, flowers blossom, fruits ripen.

You cannot escape here blessings of virtue and burnings of sin.

Here the wheel comes full circle, without stopping anywhere.

Here the oppressor's head someday rolls on the ground.

Deferred justice is referred to and applied.

Here truth always triumphs, never falsehood.

Here hatred never succeeds, love never fails.

Here if you bring light, darkness everywhere disappears.

Here there is no dogmatism except in minds of perverted men.

Here no doubt that a sword-thrust brings forth flowinng gush of warm red blood.

Again, here wounds are healed, tears are wiped, prayers are heard:

> *Here in God's world, you can die and be reborn.*

> *Here God is seen. Aye, God is verily seen!*

Where could you find, O foolish man, a better world than this world of cause and effect,

of sowing and harvesting?

> *Moreover of grace?*

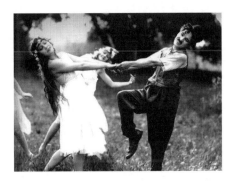

Look Death in the Face and Smile

The LifePlan

Many of our castles are built on sand. After all, loss is always going to be an inherent part of the life cycle. It gives the whole process of life meaning. Dr Elizabeth Kübler-Ross has written of the five stages of death and dying:

1 Denial and isolation

2 Anger

3 Bargaining

4 Depression

5 Acceptance.

We can see *all* of these stages in each of our daily experiences of loss, profound and trivial. Is it possible that the daily experiences of loss are actually "dry runs" designed to help teach us acceptance and good humor? Are we missing one of the great lessons of life when we chase convenience as a lifestyle?

Concentrate on what you have and not on what you have not

How quickly we manage this journey of learning, from denial to acceptance, is up to our inner attitudes and the resilience of our spirits. Are we embracing change as the agent of learning or merely spending all of our time and energy preventing loss and the growth that comes with it? Concentrate on what you have and not on what you have not. The trick to the whole game is to arrive at the stage of acceptance as quickly and painlessly as possible.

Taking care of unfinished business brings real peace. So, imagine that you find yourself with the following situation to manage. You have just undergone your full medical check-up. Your doctor calls you several days later and requests a meeting with you (and your spouse) to go over the results. You spend one of your worst weekends in recent memory as you reflect over the upcoming discussion.

During the discussion, your doctor tells you: "Well, I am very sorry to tell you this, but your results indicate that you have a terminal cancer and you have only three years to live. There will be no pain or discomfort, just a change in the overall model of your life, now drastically curtailed."

Imagine now that you have only three more years to live. Write down here, the three most important things that you would like to do with your life, if the next three years were to be your last:

1 _____

2 _____

3 _____

Now, promise yourself that you will follow through this re-prioritization of life by doing one of these three things within a month.

A LifePlan success is a game where we set goals, go for them and achieve what we set out to accomplish. Happiness is a state of mind of being satisfied with what you end up with. A LifePlan might contain the following kinds of goal:

■ get a pilot's license or get over the fear of flying;

■ learn how to control my anger;

■ learn how to be spontaneous and joyful;

■ rediscover the lost "child" within;

■ learn a musical instrument or develop an appreciation of opera;

■ go sailing around the world or just learn to sail;

■ body surf at Kuta Beach, Bali;

■ spend more quality time with my partner/children;

■ learn a martial art;

■ learn how to cook Chinese;

■ learn how to juggle, learn a language, learn how to draw;

■ get to know my spouse/kids as people.

As a physician, I was always struck by the peaceful serenity of terminally ill patients. Is it possible to be as centered as these patients without having the diagnosis of terminal disease? The definitive answer is yes! How? Be altruistically selfish: write for yourself a LifePlan.

Dr McGannon

Manage Regrets Intelligently

If only I could do it again ...

Given how short life is, are we spending our time well? Couldn't we be cramming even a little more into the time we have? Isn't there yet another ingenious way to cut finer and finer slivers of time? Are we unhappy when we cannot rush through things?

In case you have forgotten, things *do* actually take time to do properly. Some things simply can *not* be rushed; they have their own rhythm. Just go out into your garden and study it carefully. Nature will not be hurried into making roses bud or making the sky clear of clouds. Nature will, rather, make you synchronize yourself to her rhythm. The only way to know that rhythm is to study Nature (people are *part* of Nature) and realize that everybody has their own rhythm.

We go to great unnecessary lengths to get wise. What we do not always realize is that *all* the wisdom you will ever need to understand the life experience is within you already, just waiting to be discovered. By quieting the noise or internal chatter of the mind, through, say, regular meditation and prayer, the mind's eye can see clearly.

As we have all experienced, there is a sort of time lag between the actual life experience and wisdom. Do this mental exercise: When some type of change or loss happens to you, how long is the time lag until you grasp the lesson within the experience (i.e. wisdom)? (See Fig. 5.2.)

This lag, which for some can be several decades, is strictly a function of attitude. Eventually, we all "get the lesson" of every experience, sometimes six months later, sometimes six decades later. The key to a regret-free life is to get wise as early as possible by milking every experience for a lesson. When you make learning about life the career, all time becomes "your time."

In most societies today, walls are constructed to keep "them" out (and lock ourselves in): artificial boundary lines are drawn and this fortress mentality is constantly reinforced. Paradoxically, we are surprised to

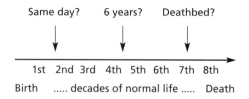

FIGURE 5.2 *Shortening the time lag to wisdom*

discover that we have unwittingly made isolation and alienation an integral part of our lives. Being stuck in this survival mode, and never learning to loosen up and let go, can be a deep source of unnecessary worry to us. If human beings are ever to have a chance to evolve from this strict survival mode of behavior to a living mode, we must learn to let go. Paradoxically, worry now is the vaccine for worry later. When we are forced back upon ourselves (death of loved one, natural disaster, car accident, air crash), we have the opportunity to re-prioritize and avoid regrets.

While coping with cancer, humorist Erma Bombeck needed an organ transplant and, even though she could have been moved to the head of the waiting list due to her prominence and wealth, she refused to do so and ultimately died of organ failure. We may be wise to take note of what this lady wrote:

IF I HAD MY LIFE TO LIVE OVER AGAIN

I would have talked less and listened more. I would have invited friends over to dinner even if the carpet was stained, or the sofa faded. I would have eaten the popcorn in the "good" living room and worried much less about the dirt when someone wanted to light a fire in the fireplace.

I would have taken the time to listen to my grandfather ramble about his youth. I would never have insisted the car windows be rolled up on a summer day because my hair had just been teased and sprayed. I would have burned the pink candle sculpted like a rose before it melted in storage.

I would have sat on the lawn with my children and not worried about grass stains. I would have cried and laughed less while watching television – and more while watching life. I would have shared more of the responsibility carried by my spouse. I would have gone to bed when I was sick instead of pretending the earth would go into a holding pattern if I weren't there for the day. I would never have bought anything just because it was practical, wouldn't show soil, or was guaranteed to last a lifetime.

Instead of wishing away nine months of pregnancy, I'd have cherished every moment and realized that the wonderment growing inside me was the only chance in life to assist God in a miracle. When my kids kissed me impetuously, I would never have said, "Later. Now go get washed up for dinner."

There would have been more "I love you's" ... more "I'm sorry" ... but mostly, given another shot at life, I would seize every minute. Look at it

*and really see it … live it … and never give it back. Stop sweating the
small stuff. Don't worry about who doesn't like you, who has more, or
who's doing what. Instead, let's cherish the relationships we have with
those who do love us. Let's think about what God HAS blessed us
with. And what we are doing each day to promote ourselves mentally,
physically, emotionally, as well as spiritually.*

*Life is too short to let it pass you by. We only have one shot at this and
then it's gone.*

I hope you all have a blessed day.

ERMA BOMBECK

Exercise: next time you feel that you are wasting your time or energy
waiting in a line or stuck in a traffic jam, take a moment to study yourself
(only boring people get bored) and your reactions to the situation. Is your
time here on earth unlimited or is it preciously short? There are no magic
weekends or vacations. Start now: realize that life itself is the real career
and you don't want to die with regrets of having missed something important to you. You do not want to look back at your life and realize that you
have missed the whole game of life because you were always absorbed by
future projects: you fell "asleep at the wheel." Life is the big career. Be
selfish. Write down now precisely what your *If I Had My Life to Live Over
Again* statement would be. Every day is full of second chances!

Managing Anger

Change the World or Change Your Mind

*The speech you make while angry will be the best speech you
ever regret.*

AMBROSE BIERCE

Do conversations or situations in your life (incompetence, inefficiency, traffic, waiting, expectations) make you angry or cynical, or distrustful or
depressed? If those are words you might use to describe your personality,
your problems will not be restricted to isolation from family and friends.
Every life situation that pulls you "off-center" and results in negative emotions will predispose you to a heart attack and stroke and, even, cancers.

Remember these key points about anger:

■ it's OK to get angry once in a while;

- know the "trigger points" for anger;
- communicate anger before it smolders into hostility;
- never make important decisions while angry;
- never eat or make love while under tension;
- unwind between work and home to prevent "overflow";
- humor is the best antidote for over-seriousness;
- living well is the best revenge – fine dining, wine tasting;
- it's not worth it;
- anger is a tempest, it will pass;
- seek distraction – a jog, a movie, go see some friends;
- communicate with your spouse/friend/partner – share the burden.

The *Bhagavad Gita*, one of Hinduism's greatest epic poems, suggests that the real battle in life has more to do with mastering our own anger and negative emotions and really nothing to do with oppression of or violence towards others. Despite the obvious setting in the *Gita* of armed kinsmen pitched against one another on a tense smoking battlefield, it really has more to do with the internal battle of right choices and self-mastery than with bloodshed and violence. The battle within the human body is for the high moral ground between "opposing moral tendencies," as Gandhi called them. This is where the real battle in life is, of course: constantly raging within us between the forces of good (truth, kindness, generosity, authenticity, impeccability, sincerity, justice, hope, humor, patience and, especially, love) and evil (greed, humorlessness, cynicism, intolerance, selfishness, laziness, ignorance, mediocrity, meanness and, especially, fear).

Thomas Merton, a man of peace and a Trappist monk, commented incisively on the *Gita* and the internal spiritual struggles of the protagonist, Arjuna:

The Gita presents a problem to some who read it in the present context of violence and war which mark the crisis of the West. The Gita appears to accept and to justify war. Arjuna is exhorted to submit his will to Krishna by going to war against his enemies, who are also his own kin, because war is his duty as a prince and as a warrior ...

The Gita is not a justification of war, nor does it propound a war-making mystique ... Arjuna has an instinctive repugnance for war and that is the chief reason why war is chosen as the example of the most repellent kind of duty. The Gita is saying that even in what appears to be most "unspiritual" one can act with pure intentions ... This consciousness itself will impose the most strict limitations on one's use of violence because that use will not be directed by one's own selfish interests, still less by cruelty, sadism and blood-lust.

THOMAS MERTON, *THE ASIAN JOURNALS*

Perhaps you cannot get rid of anger, but you can decide when to bring it out

When it comes to anger control, be realistic. Perhaps you cannot get rid of anger, but you can decide when to bring it out.

Managing Competiveness

Are You (Really) Winning the Big Game? Are You Even *In* It?

Aside from the obvious survival benefit, what is meant by "being competitive." Is it the ability to develop the skills to vanquish the opposition, to be Number One? At *what*? Who are the judges?

The father of Intuitive Breathing, Dr Leonard Orr, constructed a model of the mind by adding that there are really two aspects to this thought process: the Thinking Mind and the Proving Mind. That is, the Thinking Mind can think anything it may want and the Proving Mind will confirm that by finding data to prove that idea. The Proving Mind is the prism through which we view the world. That process takes place unconsciously and automatically all our lives.

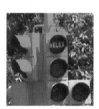

Exercise: try making the leap from road rage to road sage. Take a pause from the fast track and look at whatever you are doing throughout the day and begin to witness, in a completely non-judgemental way, these various thought files parading past our awareness. Everyone can think of modern examples of an anger-prone attitude in reaction to being kept waiting by others: of someone being late causing you real anger, only to feel stupid when the person arrives with a very compelling argument for forgiveness (death, accident, stopped to buy a gift ...).

Use your daily experiences as though they were designed to put you in touch with a part of you that needs improvement. For example, use traffic jams to generate patience and good humor. Look around in a traffic jam: people are all wrapped up in their emotions, totally lost, like lambs to the slaughter. Rise above this morass. Smile that you can find peace of mind in *any* context!

Simplify Life

Nothing to Lose, Nothing to Steal

Have you finally succeeded at complicating your life? You are not alone. What is success to you? What is the price tag of success? Must it cost so much? Success should be a natural process, the engagement of our natural talents (confusing talent and ambition results in pain) in the pursuit of meaning and fun. It is an unconscious extension of our inner bliss. Could it be simplified a little?

> *The less you have, the more you give. It seems absurd, but that is the logic of love.*
>
> MOTHER THERESA

Money: what is the role of money in your life?

Are there other currencies of success (time, fun, peak experiences)? Wealth is a poor indicator of happiness. We surround ourselves with creature comforts to the point of contradicting our genetic code. We're back to that. Our bodies and minds are simply not made to be overly pampered. You know what they say: a little material success is good, a lot is dangerous. Too much material success, and the maintenance thereof, can seriously distract us from our real mission in life. A little success is the most difficult thing in the world to have: we always want for more and we tend to overdo it. Material happiness is found somewhere in that tension between uncertainty and complete satisfaction. Appreciate what you have by "going without" for a while. If you have doubts about what you really need, set up a time when you can arrange to do without satisfying various needs. Take coffee, shopping, tobacco, drugs or sex, for example. Just observe your reaction to an electricity blackout after a storm. Without the conveniences of the lights, the heating, the cooking, the music, how do you react?

> When the ego cries at what it has lost,
> the spirit smiles at what it has gained.

With money you can buy:

■ information, but not wisdom;

■ a house but not a home;

■ a bed, but not a good night's sleep;

■ sex, but not love;

■ a clock, but not time;

■ fear, but not respect;

■ a book, but not knowledge;

■ medicine, but not health;

■ souvenirs, but not memories;

■ pleasure, but not fun;

■ contacts, but not friends;

■ blood, but not life;

■ gadgets, but not real solutions.

And, by the way, sunsets are still free.

Exercise: write this relationship on a piece of paper:

$$Happiness = \frac{Satisfaction}{Desires}$$

Even if you do not understand or agree with it, keep the piece of paper in your wallet or passport for one year. To maximize happiness, one must maximize satisfaction while keeping wants and desires to a minimum. Our happiness is directly related to satisfaction and inversely related to our desires or ambitions. Happiness increases not as the result of getting what you want (we all know the hollow feeling of finally getting that long-wanted car/house), but by being content with what you already have. Our acquisitive culture has conditioned us to believe that happiness will come once we have some material possession (the "if only" mentality). Most of anxiety comes from a mistaken belief that we are incomplete. A salesperson who has convinced you that you are incomplete without their product/service.

We are *born* complete. So there is no need to give up anything! Get rid of nothing! Give nothing away! Not necessary. Just stop acquiring! Calm the appetites that fly about our heads, which create the illusion of being incomplete.

In other words, real happiness will increase as our satisfaction with life increases and that's largely up to our perceptual skills. Happiness will also increase as our needs decrease, and this is definitely under our direct control. Either way, happiness is ours to enjoy. Otherwise, we are spending our time chasing our tails.

A Tree in the Shade of Another Cannot Grow Strong

Your children are not your children. They are the sons and daughters of Life's longing for itself. They come through you but not from you … You may give them your love but not your thoughts … You may strive to be like them, but seek not to make them like you. Life goes not backwards nor tarries with yesterday.

You are the bows from which your children as living arrows are sent forth. The Archer sees the mark upon the path of the Infinite, and He bends you with His might that his arrows may go swift and far.

KAHLIL GIBRAN

If someone told you that your children are easy to control, get your money back! Contrary to assumptions, a study from the National Institute of Mental Health (USA) found that children's health and safety concerns, choice of friends, values and school performance were all more predictive of stress symptoms than even job stress. Fathers[9] who had more concerns had more symptoms (insomnia, chest pains, fatigue, skin rashes, back pain and breathing difficulties). Men, in order to keep their health, need to take the necessary measures to ensure stable family relationships (communication, task sharing, child rearing).

When it comes to children, especially adolescents, do not do the worrying for them

When it comes to children, especially adolescents, do not do the worrying for them: that short-cuts the learning process. For them, a watchful eye and a friendly sounding board is usually all the "safety net" they want and need. Inspire confidence into them by allowing them to fight their own battles. Likewise, do your own worrying: that's your growth opportunity. However, never allow office worries to "overflow" into the home. Stop off for a workout at the gym prior to returning home or re-center yourself using the simple centering techniques described in Chapter 6.

After a moment's reflection, consider yourself a *roaring success* if you can say:

■ I did not have to give up my marriage, health or happiness to have success.

■ I can laugh heartily with my spouse on a regular basis.

- My children consider me a "friend."
- I am getting closer every day to my overall objectives in life (whatever they may be).
- I am less afraid of death (and other uncertainties) than I used to be.
- Learning to discover to live with life's paradoxes is exciting.
- Viagra-type drugs are *not* required.
- My children speak to me, without being asked.
- I have developed a tolerance for silence.
- When my partner invites me to go upstairs and make love, I do *not* have to choose between climbing the stairs and making love: I can do both.
- For me, an "all nighter" means more than not getting up to pee.
- I suffer from frequent attacks of smiling.
- Somewhere along the line I added the "what the hell …" attitude to my repertoire.
- I have developed the capacity of letting things happen, instead of trying to make them happen.
- I finally realize that in life you always get what you want, but never when you want it.
- I do not feel that I have exchanged precious years of my life, my marriage or my health for a perceived need for professional control or validation.
- I stop to smell the flowers.

Success is not getting there *first*, it is getting there without a bypass. Success is simply growing old without regrets.

Develop an Inner Toughness Against Disease

The Hardy Personality

While some people are "born tough," there are four traits of the hardy individual that we could all learn to help us to resist illness (note the similarity between the happiness characteristics and these hardy traits):

1 *Commitment*: these people are deeply self-trustful, with a sense of purpose and deep faith in their ability to make choices and commit to them wholeheartedly. Too many options can paralyze. This level of commitment brings its own energy and discipline that aids in the implementation of a strategy when under great pressure. There is nothing more powerful than a mission statement.[10]

2 *Sense of control*: hardy people take great pains to arrange their lives so that they have maximized control (especially over emotions and negative thinking) and minimized helplessness.

   What can we control? Go sit by the sea one weekend and just watch the waves tumble and crash. Hundreds of millions of tons of water are moved per second and this is many orders of magnitude less than the forces that govern and influence every variable of our lives. Call it what you will: fate, destiny, karma, the Tao, or the gigantic river of life on whose banks we nervously worry where and how the river is going. Ultimately, what we can control are the thoughts in our minds. If we have no control there, there is no control anywhere. Simpler, more down-to-earth folk could be forgiven for wondering why we just don't marvel at life and our small but significant place in it.

3 *Thirst for adventure*: these people see opportunity everywhere, constantly balancing fear of the unknown with a need to explore new things that help to enlarge their comfort zone. Failures and crises are seen not as personal threats or comments on their competence, but as lessons and opportunities for growth.

An inconvenience is an adventure wrongly understood. An adventure is an inconvenience rightly perceived.

G.K. CHESTERTON

4 *Sense of connectedness*: these people (including the religious) trust others in their lives; they have a well-developed sense of bonding to others; they feel respected.

Exercise: start from wherever you are psychologically and begin the journey of getting hardy with the first step. For example, use whatever situation around you presents itself, such as the stressful situations at work (work is the best "testing laboratory" for getting and staying centered) or overall level of fitness of your body (start by bringing your body fat down to the healthful range of 15–20%). In either event, it is the symbolic gesture of starting that counts in developing solid confidence.

Avoid Isolation Through Conspiracies

Ultimately, feeling good comes from our innate ability to forget our illusion of separation, our false loneliness, and learning how to connect with others. In learning to connect, we stop overdramatizing our lives. Our experience in the past 15 years of teaching is that these skills that enable us to feel better about our place in the world are skills that we can learn through practice.

Start with a basic fact of human existence: The whole human condition is coping with isolation at every breathing moment. Our experience of teaching thousands of business leaders and other individuals around the world is that as we learn these skills not only is our mental health improved, but our physical health as well. We have, at last, found balance! What concrete steps can we take to get closer every day to that balance?

Re-Electrify your Marriage/Partnership in Four Steps

When learning how to connect to others it is important not to forget your nearest and dearest:

1 Keep a watchful eye on those aspects of life that tend to disrupt solid marriages:
   - curiosity (spice of life, the hunt that snares the hunter);
   - boredom: lack of conspiracy/complicity/lack of depth;
   - fear of commitment;
   - getting even (revenge): stop keeping score!;
   - distance: loneliness;
   - growing apart: renew marriage vows;
   - take nothing for granted: complacency leads to arrogance – write a LifePlan;
   - ambushed by a liaison (the marriage was already wounded: betrayal is the final coup).
2 Don't keep score with a loved one:
   - learn the art of forgetting: start your life today by cleaning the slate now;
   - stop being the rescuer (or rescued);
   - try silence as a means to communicate: don't finish an argument.

3 Enchant, seduce, promote and empower:

- the art of forgetting is a natural and powerful aphrodisiac;
- make a (real) date, just like the old days;
- ask him or her when you arrive home, "And how was *your* day?";
- gently push and encourage, but only when asked;
- share what you know, but do so the way you like to learn;
- don't be afraid to say "I don't know", it's a big relief;
- surprise your mate (a tête-à-tête complete with candles, second honeymoon);
- flatter your partner by sharing the failures and the victories;
- massage, massage, massage, massage, massage;
- don't sweat the petty parts, just pet the sweaty parts.

Exercise: read this Sonnet XXIX of William Shakespeare and find how to regain and maintain this intensity of camaraderie and solace from your principal relationship. The three greatest tests that a couple can face are personal illness, old age and raising children. Use these aspects of your life to forge lasting bonds that can withstand life's caprices.

When in disgrace with fortune and men's eyes,
I all alone beweep my outcast state,
And trouble deaf heaven with my bootless cries,
And look upon myself, and curse my fate,
Wishing me like to one more rich in hope,
Featur'd like him, like him with friends possess'd,
Desiring this man's art and that man's scope,
With what I most enjoy contented least;
Yet in these thoughts myself almost despising,
Haply I think on thee, and then my state,
Like to the lark at break of day arising
From sullen earth, sings hymns at heaven's gate;
   For thy sweet love remember'd such wealth brings
   That then I scorn to change my state with kings.

4 Avoid the folly of scapegoating. To err is human. Be part of the human condition. After all, life is falling down six times and getting up seven.

Many of us are not afraid of erring, but we are deathly afraid of the losing face that comes with such a recognition of our human state. Then when our error is discovered, lies and cover-up, guilt and shame ensue and we weave a very tangled web of misrepresentations of the truth, all the time missing a unique opportunity to set up life as a no-fault proposition. Finding fault is often fruitless and counterproductive. Drop such energy-draining attitudes.

Waving your fist at your loved ones or at God serves only to confirm the presence of insecurity. An understandable psychological reflex that we all fall victim to is to point the finger when something goes wrong; the adolescent in us all comes out: "Yeah, but you did this, you said that …" and so on. It must be *someone's* fault. Why do we need to ascribe fault every time something goes wrong? Because it takes the pressure off us to do some work on *ourselves*. Ask yourself what right have we to criticize, judge or manipulate someone else. Convert your inner cynic to your inner coach.

Why should we be in such desperate haste to succeed and in such desperate enterprises? If a man does not keep pace with his companions, perhaps it is because he hears a different drummer. Let him step to the music which he hears, however measured or far away.

HENRY THOREAU

Exercise: have you ever felt out of place with the pack ? What are the benefits of being non-conformist? Could that be a good source of personal accomplishment by itself?

Make Yourself Truly (Not Just Really) Happy

Truly happy people do exist. Happiness is accessible to all: you just have to be very careful to whom you listen. Every year pharmaceutical companies are indicating that they are getting ever closer to the magic designer drugs that will balance the brain's neurotransmitters just enough to bring happiness. For those who can wait for that Pandora's Box that may be fine, but for most of us who cannot wait, what can we do at least to vanquish sadness and, if possible, achieve a sense of contentment with life?

Happiness is accessible to all: you just have to be very careful to whom you listen

During the past three decades, happiness (subjective wellbeing) has been intensely studied by researchers worldwide.[11] Here are some of the (surprising) findings:

1 *Happiness cannot be bought*: it is a generally accepted falsehood that social condition and status cause misery. If that were so, and there were a linear relationship between social status and happiness, it would stand to logic that the hyper-rich would be hyper-happy. Just not so. Although Americans earn *twice* what they did in 1957, the proportion of those reporting to researchers at the National Opinion Research Center that they were "very happy", declined from 35 to 29%. According to *Forbes* magazine, even the very rich people (who are classified as the 100 wealthiest Americans) report only a slightly greater degree of happiness over average income Americans.

   Moreover, happiness seems to defy the usual predictability: it cuts across almost all demographic lines of gender, economics, age, educational level, income and race. One of the few consistent differentials in happiness comes between married (40% happy), never-married (24% happy), and divorced people (12%).

2 *The happiness profile*: if not money, fame, nor possessions, what makes up the profile of the deeply contented person? In virtually every study, researchers have been able to identify four happy characteristics, which cascade into each other:

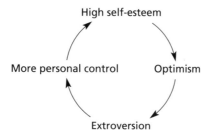

- **Self-esteem**: it all starts here – people who actually like and accept themselves feel confident about life. Contentedness with self was the best predictor of life satisfaction, more so than family life, friends and relationships. Enduring satisfaction with self is based on the self-esteem earned through self-acceptance and personal resilience.

- **Optimism**: hopeful and optimistic people (including those with an active religious faith) trust the logic of their worlds and are, as a result, not just happier, but healthier (fewer colds, flus and faster recovery from cancer and surgery). This is not blind naïve optimism but pragmatic realism. Harvard graduates found by interviews to be pessimistic in the 1940s had much less healthy profiles in the 1980s.

■ **Extroversion**: socially outgoing people tend to report more happiness and satisfaction with life and work, whether alone or in groups, than introverts. Extroverted people, armed with confidence and a sense of adventure, stride into a room wondering where their next conversation will lead them: new friends, broadened business horizons, new love.

■ **Personal control**: would you like to generate an enduring positive feeling of happiness? Regain personal control over your life – by committing to improving your time management, sleep hygiene, financial matters, health and fitness. Start by listening to the right people in your life.

3 *Happiness protects your health*: happy people, when compared to depressed people, tend to feel less hostility and are more focussed and less susceptible to diseases. Happy moments in life will provide a scientifically proven boost to your immune system, more so than the negative effects of sad or unpleasant moments. A study of middle-aged men came up with the following findings:

■ **Negative** stresses at work (destructive criticism, unrealistic deadlines, excessive workloads or conflictual relations) impact negatively on the immune system, causing colds and other infections on the day of the negative event.

■ **Positive** events (family, friends, parties, fishing, jogging – anything) actually strengthen the immune system for the next two days.[12] Surprisingly, it was a decrease in the number of positive events that more accurately predicted infection susceptibility than an increase in negative events!

So it appears that true happiness is not a function of wealth or social standing, geography, or anything external. Rather, happiness comes naturally by simply deciding to give ourselves permission to be happy. After all, this is not a rehearsal for life. If not now, when?

If No Immediate Solution Presents Itself

When faced with a worrying situation, sometimes no immediate solution presents itself and the best thing you can do is to seek distractions. Here are some suggestions:

1 After careful and complete study of the circumstances, if you can do nothing about the situation for the moment, relax, go out for a walk, go out for dinner with your spouse, have a nice bottle of wine and go to a funny movie or show. The tempest will pass. Happy moments are precious: savor them instead of putting them off.

2 Worry cold-bloodedly, free of emotional overlay. Be philosophical about the whole affair. If you are saddened by it or angered by it, the result will be emotional hand-wringing. Put it off until you have had a good run in the park or a workout at the gym. You'll be better suited for it.

3 Scribble this on to a slip of paper (business cards work fine):

> Today is the tomorrow you worried so much about yesterday –
> and all is well.

4 When all else fails, trust your genes, your brain, your companions and your inner Divinity.

TIPS FOR YOUR HEALTH ACTION PLAN

The best time to worry ... just before doing meditation or mantra

The best time to meditate ... just after worrying

The best way to jump-start a relationship ... learn to forget and start over

The best way to success ... know what you want, early to bed and rise, categorically refuse to associate with negative people

The best attitude ... life is the career: stay alert for opportunities

The best definition of success ... growing old without any regrets

The best way to confuse the enemy ... love and forgiveness

The best defence against depression ... gratitude for life's lessons

The best way to avoid jet lag ... ask "Is this trip *really* necessary?"

SELF-ASSESSMENT QUIZ

1 What are some of the most obvious symptoms of depression?
   (a) Quiet, withdrawn
   (b) Sadness
   (c) Passive

   Hint: Silence often precedes depression

2 Worrying and kids: what are the options?

(a) Worry incessantly = love
(b) Encourage, encourage, encourage
(c) To impose our views is critical

Hint: By trusting them, we learn to trust ourselves

3 What are the detrimental effects of excessive adrenaline in our blood?

(a) Increased BP
(b) Increased TGs, TC
(c) Increased platelet aggregation (thickened blood)
(d) Increased risk of strokes
(e) Increased risk of cancer

Hint: Fight-or-flight response

4 What are the detrimental effects of excessive cortisol in our blood?

(a) Increased BP
(b) Weakened immune system
(c) Increased insulin levels
(d) Increased platelet aggregation

Hint: Fight-or-flight response

5 The "hardy" profile consists of :

(a) Sense of control
(b) Fear of adventure
(c) Commitment
(d) High-intensity exercise (sprinting/squash)

Hint: Solid self-confidence

6 The same biochemical reactions occur within our bodies during physical and mental stress:

(a) True
(b) False

7 Writing a LifePlan can help you:

(a) Re-prioritize
(b) Live the present
(c) Avoid regrets
(d) Complicate your life

8 Regret is a normal part of life:

(a) True

(b) False

Hint: Regret is a waste of time

9 The following are part of the Type A profile:

(a) Anger-prone

(b) Time-urgent

(c) Good listener

10 The following are part of the Type B profile:

(a) Anger-prone

(b) Very impatient

(c) Never in a hurry

(d) Good listener

Hint: More balanced personality

Answers

1 All	**6** (a)
2 (b)	**7** (a) (b) & (c)
3 All	**8** (b)
4 All	**9** (a) & (b)
5 (a) & (c)	**10** (c) & (d)

Notes

1 Holmes, T.H., Rahe, R.H., "The social readjustment rating scale, "*Journal of Psychosomatic Research*, 1967; 11(2): 213–8.

2 If there is a Type A (aggressive. time-urgent, anger prone, all-or-nothing), there is, of course, a Type B Behavior Pattern: passive, relaxed, good at listening, contented, not frustrated, cares enough, time easy (everything in its time), easygoing. All of which leads to less adrenaline (high BP)/cortisol (prevents adrenaline breakdown) around in the blood, faster electrocardiogram responses to stress, less heart disease and, naturally, a more balanced home life. If trying to evolve into a Type B seems stressful, the other option is to understand and control the downside of the TABP, especially anger and hostility.

3 Data from angiographic studies have found that the potential for hostility (a disposition reflecting characteristics such as anger, explosive speech, cynicism and irritability) is related to the extent of the heart disease. Alternatively, further studies have demonstrated low hostility to be associated with lower heart disease and lower incidence of malignant cancers.

4 The risk factor status of TABP is supported by three prospective studies: (1) a sample of middle-aged, predominantly white-collar men employed by various firms in California (2) a population-based study of men and women in the ongoing US Framingham Study, and (3) three samples of employed men, white-collar and blue-collar, in Belgium and France (Yeung A.C. et al., *New England Journal of Medicine*, 1991; 325: 1551–6).

5 There is a downside to the unrelenting standards for high achievements, where often success is seen as a failure. Perfectionism often amounts to an excessive approval hunger, whetted at adolescence and which keeps these individuals vulnerable to criticism. They tend to avoid professional help as a sign of weakness and are more susceptible to alcoholism, depression and suicide.

6 As discussed earlier, high insulin levels promote heart disease as the result of increasing blood pressure and artery wall thickness, increased TGs and decreased HDL.

7 From the Hindu epic poem the *Bhagavad Gita*, II.3: According to Swami Vivekananda, "If one reads this one sloka – Yield not to unmanliness, O son of Pritha! It does not become you. Shake off this base faint heartedness and arise, O scorcher of foes – he gets all the merits of reading the entire *Gita*".

8 We readily accept credit for the successes and good deeds; we deserve them. Who has ever given back the undeserved winnings of a lottery? Paradoxically, despite the fact that we all recognize the growth potential of life hassles and failures, we arrange our entire existence around avoiding and, failing that, rejecting them: another lost opportunity in life's classroom. As Jack Benny once said, "I don't deserve this award, but I have arthritis and I don't deserve that either."

9 Women had the opposite profile: physical symptoms were related to job stress. They were better able to compartmentalize the family and the work demands.

10 Mission statement: this goes beyond the usual corporate offerings. A properly conceived personal mission statement is the prism through which all life events are filtered and interpreted.

11 Social scientists interviewed people to assess the impact of positive and negative feelings, mood swings and how much people smiled.

12 Daily saliva samples enabled researchers to monitor immune-surveillance by measuring antibody activity during the study.

CHAPTER SIX

WIND

▶▶▶▶▶▶▶▶▶▶▶▶▶▶▶▶▶▶▶▶▶▶▶▶▶▶▶▶▶▶▶▶▶▶▶▶▶▶

Nan-in, a Japanese master during the Meiji era (1868–1912), received a university professor who came to inquire about Zen. Nan-in served tea. He poured the visitor's cup full, and then kept on pouring. The professor watched the overflow until he could no longer restrain himself.

"It is overfull. No more will go in!"

"Like this cup," Nan-in said, "you are full of your own opinions and speculations. How can I show you Zen unless you first empty your cup?"[1]

Using the advice contained in this chapter, Mr Timebomb could:

■ find better work/life balance
■ optimize blood pressure
■ develop more stamina
■ manage work-related stress better
■ make more lucid, mistake-free decisions
■ manage crises better without panic.

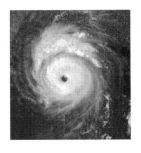

Life's Hurricanes as Tests in Themselves

Life is not *like* a hurricane, it *is* a hurricane. Looking at the image on the previous page, one can plainly see that what really matters is where you are situated during a hurricane.

If you allow yourself to be pulled off-center, away from the eye of the hurricane and into the periphery of the hurricane near the outer swirls where there is violence and destruction, you will become a cynical victim, eventually fall ill and, perhaps, not survive. No one can avoid a hurricane: they arrive uninvited in our lives and turn everything upside down. The best we can do is to manage them by getting to the center. At the center or eye of the hurricane, you will find certain new things happen to you: most immediately, you will notice a beneficial sense of detachment from life events; you will still be part of it all, but your experience will be one of peace and wonder.

In this chapter we look at the ways that most managers experience life's hurricanes, and ask the question: how do managers react to stress?

Are We Giving Ourselves Diseases?

The best way to answer that query is by looking at what is happening *inside* our bodies in response to the *outside* world. This is called biofeedback or autogenic training. Again, using our research involving some 30,000 managers, the symptoms of excessive stress they reported were consistent (see Table 6.1).

TABLE 6.1 *Symptoms of excessive stress reported by 30,000 managers (1988–2001)*

Physical symptoms	%
Chronic fatigue	80
Muscular tension	76
Sleeplessness	70
Emotional upset	70
Irritability/impatience	70
Headaches	60
Marital conflict	60
Stomach acidity	56
Emotional instability	56
Poor sleep	55
More cigarettes/alcohol	55
Sexual dysfunction	55
Anxiety, irritability	45

Psychological symptoms	%
Poor judgement	45
Spastic colon	40
Emotional withdrawal	38
Near accidents (work/driving)	36
Nervous eating	30
Nail biting/teeth grinding	27
Dry mouth/sweaty hands	25
Withdrawal, isolation	20
Chest pain	20
Spastic colon (bloating, gas, diarrhea, constipation, pain)	20
Apathy	20

What Can We Control?

If you can keep your head when all about you

Are losing theirs and blaming it on you...

If you can dream – and not make dreams your master;

If you can think – and not make thoughts your aim;

If you can meet with Triumph and Disaster

And treat those two impostors just the same.

If you can bear to hear the truth you've spoken

Twisted by knaves to make traps for fools...

Yours is the Earth and everything that's in it.

RUDYARD KIPLING, *IF*

We cannot avoid life's hurricanes (in fact, life crises perform the vital functions of decompression and cleansing); we can simply try to stay centered during the storm. We see this every day at INSEAD: successful managers do not back down from the storms of business life, they stay centered and lucid so that they can make appropriate decisions for the survival of the ship and crew. What makes the difference between success stories and failure is good mental software.

We cannot avoid life's hurricanes; we can simply try to stay centered during the storm

The experience of being centered is not reserved for anyone special and you do not need to do anything strange or weird to access this dynamic strength. We experience this every day, not just during peak experiences.

Consider the brain as a computer, with electricity, processing capabilities, memory space and so on. What interfaces the brain (hardware) with lifes storms? Surely, to have a brain is not enough, one needs the mind (software): a constantly changing constellation of feelings, attitudes, prejudices and conditioning. What are the principal tools that are used by pragmatic business people to cope with the excessive stress of their lives? Table 6.2 shows the responses of the 30,000 managers included in our research at INSEAD.

TABLE 6.2 *How do modern managers deal with excessive stress?*

Coping tools	%
Talk to someone	72
Tough it out	58
Reading	58
More cigarettes/alcohol	55
Go for a walk	45
Exercise	45
Prayer	32
Visualization	21
Take a pill	21
Massage	20
Deep breathing	20
Meditate	17
Play with the children	17
Avoid the issue, escape	12

There is certainly no shortage of techniques and insights on the subject of mind control. Presented here are the diverse techniques that many thousands of international managers report to us as effective in the fast-track life of business.

Develop an Appreciation for Silence

A Real Refuge from the Background Noise

We borrow here from one of our most insightful writers of the 20th century, Aldous Huxley:

The twentieth century is, among other things, the Age of Noise. Physical noise, mental noise and noise of desire – we hold history's

*record of them. And no wonder; for all the resources of our almost
miraculous technology have been thrown into the current assault
against silence. That most popular and influential of all recent
inventions, the radio, is nothing but a conduit through which pre-
fabricated din can flow into our homes. And this din goes far deeper,
of course, than the eardrums. It penetrates the mind, filling it with a
Babel of distractions, blasts of corybantic or sentimental music,
continually repeated doses of drama that brings no catharsis, but
usually creates a craving for daily or even hourly emotional enemas.*

*And where, as in most countries, the broadcasting stations support
themselves by selling time to advertisers, the noise is carried from the
ear, through the realm of phantasy, knowledge and feeling to the
ego's core of wish and desire. Spoken or printed, broadcast over ether
or wood pulp, all advertising copy has but one purpose – to prevent
the will from ever achieving silence. Desirelessness is the condition of
deliverance and illumination. The condition of an expanding and
technologically progressive system of mass production is universal
craving. Advertising is the organized effort to extend and intensify the
workings of that force, which (as all the saints and teachers of all the
higher religions have always taught) is the principal cause of suffering
and wrongdoing and the greatest obstacle between the human soul
and its Divine Ground.*

ALDOUS HUXLEY, "ON SILENCE" 1946

People tend to find silence uncomfortable because it represents a pregnant pause in the incessant chatter that makes us more robotic and less
spontaneous. Try entering the silence in these ways:

1 *Active listening with new ears*: the main reason why people complain
  about memory problems is that they are talking when they should be
  listening. Type A people are particularly poor at active listening as they
  often finish other people's sentences with their own words.
  Exercise: study yourself at any social function such as a cocktail
  party and the truth will be revealed – when introduced to a stranger,
  we can be so eager to hear the way that our name is pronounced
  upon presentation to the stranger that we do not hear the name of the
  stranger and then think that our memory is shot.

2 *Talking moratorium*: for once, let the others speak. Don't worry, they
  will. The reasons why people go to retreats or ashrams are not just
  related to the substance of the weekend, but also the structure: certain
  collective conventions must be observed and all individual needs are

subserved to the group's needs. If you cannot learn sign language or use a pad to communicate basic ideas, try to go just three hours without hearing your voice. Impossible? Try merely *listening* at dinner this weekend.

Never Panic in a Crisis

Everything Is Under Control

In the end, after all, in exchange for the pain caused us by certain crises, come valuable lessons. Study the Chinese character for the concept of "crisis":

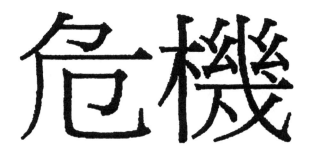

Within this character are two separate, though intertwined, characters: (1) danger, hence, caution; and (2) hidden opportunity. *That's* the mindset to work towards – it's a good idea to recognize the inherent danger in change and to protect yourself from the imminent and real dangers (as opposed to the imagined sort) while keeping a keen eye on whatever hidden opportunity might be waiting for us within.

> Do not fear the winds of adversity.
> A kite rises against the wind, rather than with it.

Worry in the form of concern that leads to planning is appropriate. Worry in the form of panic that leads to paralysis is the beginning of the downward spiral. Acute anxiety (panic) attacks do not just happen. They are the result of smoldering problems and poor mental discipline. When struck by a panic attack (such as just before a meeting, conference or doctor's appointment) try these simple steps:

- Using your natural breathing, bring your mind over the center of your hurricane.
- Wait, do not speak or decide anything critical until these signs of lucidity appear: thoughts/voices slowing down, then, slowed breathing, a sense of detachment (feeling of distance from the event), then a smile. Once calm, the mind will start its survival/problem-solving mania, what it does best, with emotional overlay.
- Ask: what are the facts?
- Set a time limit, write a temporary Action Plan (an Action Plan may include asking your spouse for advice, or collecting more information).
- Once calm, and the dust of the first Action Plan has settled, reassess the fallout.

Anxiety is often accompanied by such physical symptoms as heart palpitations, shortness of breath, hyperventilation, muscle tension in the back and neck, excessive sweating, dry mouth, dizziness or nausea. Other steps that can help with anxiety include the elimination of caffeine, alcohol and sugar; a good diet; a good multiple vitamin-mineral supplement; regular exercise; stress-reduction techniques such as breathing, relaxation and meditation; counseling; time management; and effective communication skills.

Detoxify the Mind with a Sense of Humor

> *A merry heart doeth good like a medicine; but a broken spirit drieth the bones.*
>
> PROVERBS 17:22

Excessive pressure, particularly when it is self-imposed, leads to high blood pressure, muscle tension, immunosuppression, headaches, depression, heart disease, and possibly cancer. Excessive seriousness indicates that something is being protected or hidden within: we are afraid of taking off the mask. We put on the guardsman mask to convey a weighty importance commensurate with our position or task at hand. A doctor delivering dire news in a comical way is inappropriate.

During mirthful laughter, the mind provides to the body benefits that are numerous and enduring (see Table 6.3).

TABLE 6.3 *Physical effects of laughter on the body*

Body area affected	Physical effect
Heart and lungs	Lowers BP Increases vascular blood flow
Nervous system	Decreases pain perception

Hormonal[2]	Decreases blood levels of stress chemicals:
	    Beta endorphin
	    Corticotrophin
	    Cortisol
	    Growth hormone
	    Prolactin
	    Adrenaline compounds

Immunologic system	Decreases blood levels of immuno-suppressive chemicals:
	    Cortisol
	    Adrenaline compounds
	Increases activity of Natural Killer (NK) cells
	    (NK cells fight tumor cells)
	Increases interferon gamma activity (IFN), which
	    activates NK, T and B cells and immunoglobulins
	Increases salivary IgA, which protects the
	    respiratory tract against infectious invaders

Muscular	Tones the diaphragm and accessory respiratory muscles
Respiratory	Increases O_2 to the muscles Laughing, coughing and hiccoughing help to clear airways of mucus

There are also some beneficial psychological effects of laughter:

- Laughter is cathartic: it allows pent-up tension to be released.
- Shameless hamming (such as a stand-up comic or performing karaoke) is an excellent tool to build confidence and control the ego.
- Laughter helps us temporarily to forget anger and fear, the first step to reconciliation.
- Laughter provides the opportunity of starting over: a "reset button" after a long hard day.
- Laughter can, by helping us to detach from a stressful situation, create a feeling of power and hope.

If you can laugh at it, you can survive it.

BILL COSBY

An intriguing study presented at the American Heart Association's Scientific Sessions in 2000 confirmed what we have already said – one of the most effective ways to protect the heart and brain from arteriosclerosis is to laugh hard and often. Results of this study showed that heart patients were 40% less likely than their healthy counterparts to laugh at a variety of life situations. It appears that using laughter as a coping mechanism helps to decrease hostility and encourages us not to take ourselves so seriously.

One of the most effective ways to protect the heart and brain from arteriosclerosis is to laugh hard and often

Alternatively, in a study of people aged 65 and over who were initially free of heart disease, researchers found that those feeling symptoms of depression (fear, loneliness, irritability, low concentration, sleeplessness) were 40% more likely to develop heart disease.

Not every situation requires a head-first serious approach: heads get cracked that way. A moment's reflection will often allow you to gain the nimble lucidity required to see what role to play from one moment to the next. Take the humorous approach. Enjoy witnessing your intelligence curve cross your wisdom curve. Laughter can prevent an event being overdramatized.

> Make it your dead serious business to laugh hard and often to counterbalence life's nay-sayers and worry-mongers. There is absolutely no better revenge.

Exercise: using a mirror, do a mock presentation of yourself to a new acquaintance. Examine your face when you are speaking: how often do you smile? Do you convey a sense of comfort or constraint? Can you see the power of a smile? A smile, when sincere, is the best single shield of protection against the pervasive negativity that surrounds us every day. Then, make a conscious effort to bring a little smile to every encounter you have at the office and home for just a week. Note the changes, both in terms of the reactions of peers and family members and in terms of how you see the world. No one can explain it to us, but putting on a smile will definitely advance your life and career in the right direction.

Instead of poisoning the home front after a conflictual day, spare the family the melodrama of your day and arrive at home with several humorous stories and laughter. That is how they will remember you!

Deep Breathing

Change the World or Change Your Mind

> Don't be dishonest to your vital breath; worship that
> only, abide in that only, accept it as yourself.
>
> NISARGARDATTA MAHARAJ

As goes the mind so goes the breathing pattern. Our breathing pattern (and resting heart rate) can act as excellent barometers for how centered our minds are.

At times when you're feeling particularly stressed to the point of hyperventilating, force yourself to breathe slowly and deeply. If your breathing has become shallow and rapid, this results in trapping CO_2 in the base of the lungs. CO_2 trapping by itself can give you a subjective feeling of anxiety. So, before the big presentation, pull off the fast track, take five deep breaths to blow off the CO_2, and infuse the blood with O_2. That way you have the added edge of being centered.

One-Minute Deep Breathing Programs

> Two months without food
> Two weeks without water
> A few minutes without air.

The following deep breathing programme can act as a form of reset button for the mind in crisis.

While standing

Try this breathing program while you are standing (while waiting in line, for example):

- Relax your facial muscles, don't clench your teeth, drop your shoulders and take a nice deep breath, through your nose.
- Inhale first with your belly (to fill out the lower parts of your lungs), then continue to inhale with your upper chest (to fill out the upper parts of your lungs).

- Now exhale all at once, completely, in order to get rid of the CO_2 trapped in the base of your lungs. By itself, blowing off CO_2 will produce a warm sense of alert relaxation.

- Acknowledge your thoughts, feelings and emotions as you inhale and then release whatever tension is created by them as you exhale. Stay clear headed and calm.

- Repeat with your eyes closed three times or until your mind is quiet and focussed.

While seated

Try this breathing program while you are seated (while in a waiting room, for example):

- Slip your shoes off and place your feet on the floor. Sit up straight and tall, distributing your weight evenly on both hip bones. Rest your arms on your thighs.

- Relax your facial muscles, don't clench your teeth, swallow a few times to make sure that your throat is relaxed.

- Inhale first with your belly (to fill out the lower parts of your lungs), then continue to inhale with your upper chest (to fill out the upper parts of your lungs).

- Now exhale all at once, completely, in order to get rid of the CO_2 trapped in the base of your lungs. By itself, blowing off CO_2 will produce a warm sense of alert relaxation.

- Acknowledge your thoughts, feelings and emotions as you inhale and then release whatever tension is created by them as you exhale. Stay clear headed and calm.

- Repeat with your eyes closed three times or until your mind is quiet and focussed.

- Open your eyes and put a smile on your face.

Alternate nostril breathing

This breathing program is perfect for energizing your brain after a long morning. Although it sounds a little weird, it's a very powerful technique for calming yourself during times of intense stress. It is just another breathing technique that can help you clear your mind and control the noise of your thoughts in just *2 minutes*. Try it out:

- If you are in your office, tell your secretary not to disturb you for the next 3 minutes (always give yourself a couple of minutes margin), no phone calls, no interruptions.

- Sit upright with your spine erect and your head straight but relaxed.

- Use your right hand for the exercise. Your thumb will control your right nostril and your index finger will control your left nostril.

- Close the right nostril with the thumb and inhale slowly and fully through the left nostril.

- Hold your breath for 2 or 3 seconds only, *no longer*.

- Close the left nostril with your index finger and exhale slowly through the right nostril.

- Inhale through the *same* right nostril while the left nostril is still closed.

- Again hold your breath for a few seconds only.

- Close the right nostril and exhale through the left nostril. This completes one round. Complete three rounds and observe.

- When you are ready, open your eyes very slowly, stretch your neck, arms and hands.

- When you want, stand up and stretch your spine backward very slowly, while resting your hands on your lower back.

- Repeat the whole process for about 60 seconds, and you'll feel like (because you will be) a new person. Now you are ready to continue your day with more positive energy.

Self-Enquiry

What Am I Anyway?

Just as proper nutrition is essential to our body's health and survival, so do we also need to monitor carefully our "foods for thought" to ensure the proper working of our brain. Allowing our minds to become polluted with certain, less than desirable values could lead not only to poorer physical health, but also to mental weakness.

Take, for example, the so-called "youth-obsessed culture," coming primarily from the USA (and within the USA from Hollywood), but willingly accepted and even paid for by European and Asian cultures. You can see the subliminal, yet "in-your-face" messages on the TV and in the newspapers every day:

- "You are never too rich or too thin."
- "No pain, no gain."
- "Just do it."

- "Whatever it takes…"
- "Lead, follow, or get the hell out…"
- "Wealth can buy health."
- "Time is money."

In this youth-obsessed culture, we are asked to pay excessive attention to only one aspect of our life – our body's look – at the expense of the more lasting transcendent aspects (raw vitality, values, the intellect, literature, family, spirituality, poetry and so on) with the obvious results, which resemble Huxley's *Brave New World*:

- Plastic surgery, to handle our well-deserved wrinkles, is becoming ever more popular.
- Charlatans remove our fat tissue with diet pills (diet pills are weaker cousins of "speed," which ruins our hearts and brains) and liposuction (depriving us of family walks).
- Children are killing children.
- The wise people of our culture (the aged) are sequestered in retirement homes.
- We imitate TV/movie stars and corrupt athletes: life imitating so-called "art."
- Minors and retarded people are condemned to capital punishment.
- We eat food made by machines, thousands of kilometers away.

Exercise: if some stranger presented himself at your front door, asking if he could speak about his values to your children, clearly you would forcibly reject his offer. And yet, we allow such strangers in every day: it is called TV. We actually *pay* for it to be pumped into our house, like a silent visitor, there to ***TV is a dangerous babysitter*** reprogram our children, steadily undoing everything we have worked so hard for all these years. TV is a dangerous babysitter. *Do a TV moratorium for a week*: pull the antenna and watch the reaction of your family.

> Karl Marx said that religion is the opiate of the people. If he were alive today, he would have replaced "religion" with "TV."

What follows are four classic texts from the world's literature, all proposing alternative approaches to couterbalance the largely negative deluge from the youth-obsessed culture.

1   *The One remains, the many change and pass;*

Heaven's light forever shines, Earth's shadows fly;

Life, like a dome of many-coloured glass,

Stains the white radiance of Eternity,

Until Death tramples it to fragments. – Die,

If thou wouldst be with that which thou dost seek!

Follow where all is fled! – Rome's azure sky,

Flowers, ruins, statues, music, words, are weak

The glory they transfuse with fitting truth to speak.

PERCY BYSSHE SHELLEY,

ADONAIS: AN ELEGY ON THE DEATH OF JOHN KEATS

2   In Huxley's *Divine Ground*, he presents four general principles as the cornerstones of his Perennial Philosophy:

> *First, the phenomenal world of matter and of individual consciousness – the world of things and animals and men and even gods – in a manifestation of a Divine Ground within which all partial realities have their beings, and apart from which they would be nonexistent.*
>
> *Second: human beings are capable not merely of knowing about the Divine Ground by inference; they can realize its existence by direct intuition, superior to discursive reasoning. This immediate knowledge unites the knower with that which is known.*
>
> *Third: man possesses a double nature, a phenomenal ego and an eternal Self, which is the inner man, the spirit, the spark of divinity within the soul. It is possible for a man, if he so desires, to identify himself with the spirit and therefore with the Divine Ground, which is of the same or like nature with the spirit.*
>
> *Fourth: man's life on earth has only one end and purpose: to identify himself with his eternal Self and so to come to unitive knowledge of the Divine Ground.*

3 The Hindu sacred text *Katha Upanishad*, in which Nachiketas searches for (and solves) the mystery of Life and Death:

Know the Self (Atman) as Lord of the chariot;

and the body as the chariot itself,

Know the intellect (reason) as the charioteer,

and the mind indeed is the reins.

The horses, they say, are the senses;

Objects of the senses (selfish attachments) are the paths they travel.

He who has not the right understanding and whose mind is never steady

is not the rule of his life, like a bad driver with wild horses.

But he who has the right understanding and whose mind is ever steady

is the ruler of his life, like a good driver with well–trained horses.

The man whose chariot is driven by reason, who watches and

holds the reins of his mind, reaches the End of his journey, the supreme

everlasting Spirit.[3]

In this metaphor, nothing is served by the stoic renunciation wherein our horses (the senses) should be subjugated to a severe deprivational and puritanical mindset. More intelligently, the sense and our desires (which give us life energy and vitality) should be trained and channeled to achieve our objectives in life. So many of us have failed to forge the balance between our head and our heart.

In one case, our head (the intellect or charioteer, above) dominates the senses and desires and we have no driving passion in life because the horses are too crushed to get us through. At the other end of the spectrum, the desires or senses are too strong (uncontrolled horses) and our ability to decide the best way becomes veiled in longing.

4 *All the world's a stage,*

  And all the men and women merely players:

  They have their exits and their entrances;

  And one man in his time plays many parts,

  His act being seven ages. At, first the infant,

  Mewling and puking in the nurse's arms.

  Then the whining schoolboy, with his satchel

  And shining morning face, creeping like a snail

  Unwillingly to school. And then the lover,

  Sighing like a furnace, with a woeful ballad

  Made to his mistress' eyebrow. Then a soldier,

  Full of strange oaths, and bearded like the pard,

  Jealous in honour, sudden and quick in quarrel,

  Seeking the bubble reputation

  Even in the cannon's mouth. And then the justice,

  In fair round belly with good capon lined,

  With eyes severe and beard of formal cut,

  Full of wise saws and modern instances;

  And so he plays his part. The sixth age shifts

  Into a lean and slippered pantaloon,

  With spectacle on nose and pouch on side;

  His youthful hose, well saved, a world too wide

  For his shrunk shank; and his big manly voice,

  Turning again towards childish treble, pipes

  And whistles in his sound. Last scene of all,

  That ends this strange and eventful history,

  In second childishness and mere oblivion,

  Sans teeth, sans eyes, sans taste, sans every thing.

WILLIAM SHAKESPEARE, *AS YOU LIKE IT*, ACT II, SCENE VII

If we pay too much attention to the state of our body, as our body ages, we invite misery. If we concentrate on the other aspects of life, the aging process becomes a journey of fearless discovery. Enduring happiness comes from playing the detached game of mastery of the desires and the intellect in a dynamic tension. Such mastery can be accomplished through meditation.

Meditation: Polishing the Mirror

There is plenty of wisdom all around us; even without going into a library or a temple: wisdom surrounds us. However, living in a sort of collective hypnosis, we find it so very difficult to recognize. In many ways we are like philosophical street beggars sitting on top of a mountain of gold.

What is meditation?

Meditation is an invitation to understand the inner forces that influence our thinking processes and, in turn, our decisions and our lives. Through meditation, we can remove the stains of pride, anger and fear that prevent us from reflecting on this cosmic wisdom. It is done through the development of the "witness" within. The witness can detach itself from the incessant "thought parade."

What exactly is meditation then and what is it not?

Meditation is an invitation to understand the inner forces that influence our thinking processes and, in turn, our decisions and our lives

Meditation:

- Is a safe and highly effective tool (one-pointed concentration).
- Is a tuning in to states of detached awareness.
- Is a pragmatic, portable way to control our thought parade and emotions.
- Is a refuge from negative, neurotic thoughts that lead to panic.
- Can help distinguish real from imaginary problems.
- Creates space, centers the mind, and allows you to witness the workings of the Thought Parade.

Meditation is not:

- A state of stupor, sleep, or drowsiness.
- A loss of consciousness or control.
- Time/labor intensive.

- An escape from life.
- Effective unless we can listen to the inner voice.

Table 6.4 shows the different stages of meditation.

TABLE 6.4 *Stages of meditation*

Stage	Sign
Better breathing control	Awareness of conditioned behavior; possible discomfort from negative thoughts yet unmastered
Better control of thought parade	Judging-mind/emotions observed
Physiology control	Normalized blood pressure, pulse, breathing and better sleep
Detached awareness	Observation without commentary, freedom from conditioning/habits[4]
Be here now[5]	Fulfilling self-potential

How and When to Meditate

Practice makes permanent
Perfect practice makes perfect.

AL WOODS (TIGER'S FATHER)

Meditation is best practiced with regularity. Start with 3 minutes in the morning, upon arising, to gain control of your thoughts, and do another 3 minutes in the evening before sleep, to "switch off."

- Sit as comfortably as possible in your chair, feet flat on the floor, back straight, but relaxed. Ideally, at first, you will want to seek out a quiet corner to minimize distractions. As you become more proficient, it will not matter where you are.
- Then, rest your hands on your laps or knees, drop your shoulders and breathe slowly and deeply until you have focussed on the natural wavelike aspect of your breathing, as if you were listening to the waves of the sea, "breathing" on to the beach, in...out...in...out...and so on.
- Now, while allowing these breathing waves to continue, imagine yourself in a movie theatre, watching not a film, but your own thoughts parading on the stage, as though they were animated characters. This is your "thought parade." View your thoughts as

uninvited guests, parading across your stage. As your thoughts prance and strut in front of you trying to get your attention away from your breathing, do not allow yourself to be overly distracted or enchanted by them. The thought parade is the sideshow, the main attraction is your breathing.

■ "Gently but firmly": remember these words. Just as with children, as your various thoughts arise, don't fight with them. Acknowledge them and allow them to move on. When the thoughts are distracting you, *gently but firmly* bring your attention back to the wavelike aspect of your breathing. This is the start of developing mental discipline: thought control. Liberation from the constant pummeling from negative thoughts going by is at hand…

■ Just let go and drift for a change…

Now, the hurricanes of our lives and in our minds have become more manageable.Throughout daily life, even when not meditating, remember: *gently but firmly.*

What to Expect

Meditation will not bring fancy hallucinations into your life, nor talking to God or anything like that. In fact, over time, you will notice that nothing really happens: anger doesn't happen, nor depression, nor blood pressure. If it is thrills you are seeking, go bungee jumping after writing a LifePlan. A typical response of a manager practicing a 3-minute meditation regime for only a couple of weeks, is as follows: "Having practiced for about six months now, I can say that I have been able to develop a distinct sense of detachment, as though I had new eyes."

Peace of mind

Before speaking or making any critical decisions, use your breathing to bring your mind over the center of the hurricane. You will know if your mind has been stabilized over the eye of the hurricane if you start experiencing the symptoms of peace of mind. When asked to report subjective or objective signs induced by a daily 3–4-minute meditation, participants in our Health Management Program listed the following findings:

■ An inability to worry for no good reason (which some may find a good reason to worry!).

■ No more scapegoating, criticizing or judging others.

■ A palpable sense of completeness, of no wanting or lacking.

- An enduring sense of humor, in *all* situations.
- A higher anger threshold: getting angry less, staying angry less.
- Freedom from time obsession, often confused with disorientation.
- Observation without commentary, freedom from conditioning/ habits.
- A realization that you are pretty complete, and not really in need of being saved.
- Intense enjoyment in letting things happen and just witnessing them …
- A realization that the world is not so bad after all, deserving of our acceptance.
- The loss of the fanatical need to control everything, from the weather to people in our lives.
- An irrepressible desire to converse with children.

You will find that once you have stated to rewrite your mind's software, there will most certainly be perceptible changes. Keep an eye open for these changes, as they represent the peace of mind that comes with the detachment that regular meditation brings.

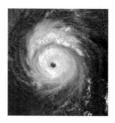

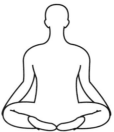

FIGURE 6.1 *Staying centered makes life's hurricanes manageable*

Mantra: an Antioxidant for the Mind?

When I first heard of meditation and mantra, it was as part of a senior management seminar, which had a component on health management offered to a group of 25 managers. After a brief overview of the practice, we were asked to slip off our shoes and unroll a large towel to sit on. I just hummed as my mantra and found that after just 5 minutes of eyes closed with mantra, I felt a natural joy overcome me and the sensation lasted until the next morning. Upon awakening, I felt the feeling had worn off but returned immediatly after doing mantra for 3 minutes. That was five years ago and I have done this brief, but highly effective, technique nearly every morning since then.

SENIOR MANAGER

What is Mantra?

Mantra is the use of a repeated phrase to abolish or curb wandering thought, and as such mantra is a powerful centering device.

The human soul of every human being constantly yearns for contact with something far greater – call it the collective consciousness – than the mere limits of the individual. Mantra can act as the bridge between the local and the universal.

The faculty of voluntarily bringing back a wandering attention over and over again is the very root of judgment, character and will. An education which should include this faculty would be the education par excellence.

WILLIAM JAMES, PSYCHOLOGIST

Is Mantra for You?

Only you can tell. If your livelihood depends on how quickly you process information, the chances are excellent that you are already using a mantra without even knowing the consequences. If your days are filled with endless streams of thoughts (both negative and positive), punctuated by occasional bouts of boredom, mantra will help regain control over the thought parade, before negative thinking can establish a beachhead.

While mantras are usually assigned to you by a spiritual leader (guru), you may well already have a mantra, probably developed during adolescence or early adult life. If it includes:

- "If only life could be like…"
- "I'll never make it."
- "Oh shit, another change to get used to."
- "I'll be destitute if I don't steal or lie."
- "I don't deserve success."
- "She hates me."
- "Life's just one hassle after another."
- "I would be happy if only…"
- "Why me?"
- "Life is very unfair."

Ask yourself, where have these mindsets got you?

Then, try one of the many time-honored substitutes that are in existance. Set your mood through your choice of daily mantras (go beyond the conscious mind). Remember, these are completely secular tools used to center your mind, they have no religious affiliation whatsoever. Whatever mantra you use, realize that it is of little importance whether you actually understand the words. The mind is concentrating on the long, melodious exhalation while humming it and this, by itself, disciplines the mind and controls negative thinking.

Some alternative mantras are as follows:

- **Humming breathing**: this is an excellent mantra-like technique ("hummmm" sound while exhaling) to use while waiting for traffic lights to change to green, or anywhere you can have a few minutes privacy.

  Sit comfortably with your neck and shoulder muscles relaxed; inhale deeply. Exhale slowly singing the word "hum" on one note; hold the m sound as you continue to exhale. Try to keep the tone steady and resonant until complete exhalation. Then, take another deep breath and start again. Repeat five times.

  Note: choose a pitch that is comfortable for your voice. Try not to let the sound die down at the end: push a little harder to keep a resonant tone until complete exhalation.

- "There are no problems, just opportunities."

- **Om** (pronounced OHM): this is a tried and true mantra, the grand-daddy of them all, used with extraordinary success for thousands of years as a centering device for the mind. As a monosyllabic mantra, you could also use "love," "one" or simply hum and try to extend the exhalation as long as possible. As you hum the mantra, feel your whole body vibrate as if the mantra was massaging your inner parts.

■ For those who like to know the meaning of their mantra:

> Lead me from the Unreal to the Real
> Lead me from the Darkness into Light
> Lead me from Death into Immortality.[6]

■ **The Gayatri mantra**: this mantra will improve the way your intellect
works in crises:

> *Om Bhur Bhva Svah*
> *Om Tat Savitur Varenyam Bhargo*
> *Devasya dimahi, di yoyona prachodayad*
> *Om*

RG VEDA 3, 62

Exercise: use the real world as your laboratory. As other senior managers have done, give yourself permission to try out less conventional
techniques that have been around for many thousands of years. Choose a
mantra from above, use it when you are alone in your car and then
observe the quietness of your mind when you arrive at your destination.
You already know how to rush; do you know how to wait?

The Fine Art of Letting Go

He who binds to him a joy,

Doth that wingèd life destroy.

But he who kisses that joy as it flies,

Lives in eternity's sunrise.

WILLIAM BLAKE, *ETERNITY*

For a Change Enjoy the View from the Back of the Bus

Follow-up research into the efficient management of anger and the entire
Type A Behavior Pattern (TABP) has yielded some very positive news for us
Type A go-getters: after a year of work on anger management, heart patients
were able to reduce episodes of heart attacks by 60%.

One of the biggest challenges for smart people is to find out which experiences require an *active* "jump in with both feet" approach and which

experiences require a *passive* "let it be" approach. The vital importance of not trying to control, of not straining, is illustrated in the physiology of your own body (see Table 6.5).

Learning to go "with the flow" or roll with the punches would also enable us to gradually shift from the status of a *victim* of circumstance (here the attitude is judgemental) to the *witness* state: a more open state of mere appreciation of life' s maddingly cryptic methods. All the time keeping our sense of humor and confidence intact to live another day. Save your "big guns" for the really important issues. Practise serenity; it will come in handy someday.

TABLE 6.5 *The effects of straining/excess control on natural bodily functions*

Natural bodily functions	The effects of excess control
Eating	Indigestion, constipation, obesity
Defecation	Hemorrhoids, bleeding
Urination	Pain
Childbirth	Complications, pain
Sexual expression	Impotence, frigidity, isolation
Sleeping	Insomnia

What did Blake mean by kissing that joy as it flies? Need we possess the experience to appreciate it or can we simply extract the pleasure as it passes? Leasing, as a philosophy, is cheaper and more condusive to staying free of the fetters of ownership. Can you appreciate the flowers without actually picking them?

All primates tend to cling, especially during moments of anxiety. We have all seen the zoo chimp separated from its mother clinging to a surrogate piece of woolen rug. Are we any better? We humans look at everything and everyone in our lives through the prism of our needs.

Embrace and welcome every experience as is. To determine your role (if any) in it, first quiet the mind through meditation, then listen to the internal voice to find the clear path. Have confidence in the voice and be unafraid to deal with the lessons that the consequences bring.

Finally, refuse to move on to the next experience without having extracted every bit of wisdom possible. The difference between wise living and foolish living lies within. Do the best you can and then let go of it. Having done that, understanding and wisdom can seep in slowly.

When No Other Refuge Works, Find God

Of our 30,000 database of managers, 32% reported that they subscribed to the use of prayer to find refuge and solace from the incessant stresses of business life. Knowing managers as well as we do, this did not surprise us for two reasons: (1) managers are first of all human beings with a heart and blood, and (2) managers are *practical*. They are after solutions to real stress and have little time to waste.

No one is beyond prayer's benefits. True to its reputation, the modern business community is an extremely pragmatic, efficient, no-nonsense group of highly individualistic people. A less well-known or appreciated fact is that to "get the job done" the modern manager is rediscovering traditional methods of alleviating excessive stress, such as mind centering with

No one is beyond prayer's benefits

mantra, meditation and prayer. Whatever your cultural background, a cursory look back over our lives confirms the true solace to be found in communicating with the Infinite, however secular or religious, however cynical or open-minded, however agnostic or devout.

At the end of the day, if we create our worries as the result of an undisciplined mind, then we must seek inner advice as one of the most effective antidotes to profound stress and anxiety. Does faith work? It works for those whose sincere search for competent counsel is accompanied by a willingness to work hard at implementing any advice given. As your self-trust increases, your trust in life's process also grows and you may notice a deep yearning for knowing what forces are operative behind the Grand Design of life.

An Executive's Prayer Book

Here are some sublime examples of the kind of extracts/prayers a busy executive could collect together in a "prayer book." It is, in fact, a compilation of favorites sent to us over the years.

1 *A story:*
   One night a man had a dream. He dreamed that he was walking along a beach with God. Across the sky, he saw scenes from life flashed before him. For each scene, he noted two sets of footprints in the sand, his own and that of God. When the last scene of his life flashed before him, he looked back at the trail of footprints. He noticed that many times along the path of his life, especially during the toughest

and saddest moments, there was only one set of footprints. Confused by this, he confronted God: "God, you said to me that once I decided to follow you, you would walk with me all the way. But what I see now is that during the most challenging parts of my life, there is only one set of footprints. I do not understand: when I needed you most, you seem to abandon me."

"My dear precious child," God replied, "I love you deeply and would never abandon you. During those times of trial and tribulation, when you see only one set of footprints, it was then that I was carrying you."

FOOTPRINTS (AUTHOR UNKNOWN)

2 Lord, I know not what I ought to ask of thee; Thou only knowest what I need. Thou loves me better than I know to love myself. O Father, give to Thy child that which he himself knows not how to ask. I dare not ask either for crosses or for consolations. I simply present myself before thee, I open my heart to Thee. Behold my needs which I know not myself, see and do according to Thy tender mercy. Smite or heal, depress me or raise me up. I adore all Thy purposes without knowing them. I am silent; I offer myself as sacrifice. I yield myself to Thee; I would have no other desire than to accomplish Thy will. Teach me to pray. Pray thyself in me. Amen.

FRANÇOIS DE SALIGNAC FENELON,
ARCHBISHOP OF CAMBRAY, 1651–1715,

3 Do not stand at my grave and weep, I am not there, I do not sleep.

I am a thousand winds that blow; I am the diamond glint in the snow.

I am the sunlight in the unripened grain, I am the gentle autumn rain.

When you awaken in the morning hush, I am the swift uplifting rush

Of quiet birds encircling flight.

I am the soft stars that shine at night.

Do not stand at my grave and weep, I am not there, I did not die.

4 Lead me from the Unreal to the Real

Lead me from the Darkness into Light

Lead me from Death into Immortality

...and I shall follow without hesitation.

5 *O Lord, make me an instrument of Thy peace.*

Where there is hatred, let me sow love;

Where there is injury, pardon;

Where there is doubt, faith;

Where there is despair, hope;

Where there is darkness, light;

And where there is sadness, joy.

O Divine Master, grant that I may not so much seek to be consoled, as

to console;

To be understood, as to understand;

To be loved, as to love;

For it is in giving that we receive

It is in pardoning that we are pardoned;

And it is in dying that we are born to Eternal Life.

ST FRANCIS OF ASSISI

TIPS FOR YOUR HEALTH ACTION PLAN

The best time to laugh ... when you are afraid or hurt

The best way to keep from crying ... laugh

The best way to get to sleep after a stressful day ... repeat at bed-time: I have done my best, now I shall take my deserved rest; may the morning sunshine bring answers to my worries

The best stimulant for the brain ... oxygen

The best mind/body workout ... yoga

The best path to serenity ... daily meditation

The best way to tie up loose ends ... write a lifeplan

The best mantra ... "Thank you" 25 times on arising and going to sleep

The best way to let go ... humor

Frequently Asked Questions

Stress, Coping and Personality

Q When should I **meditate**? How much is enough? What should I expect?

■ Upon arising, do a 3-minute meditation to center the mind. In general, do meditation as long as it takes you to smile widely and promise yourself that *nobody* at the office or home will pull you "off-center."

Q. Are **Type As** mentally tougher?

■ When challenged, research shows that Type As have higher adrenaline and cortisol levels and, in fact, recover more slowly than Type Bs. The key to coping appears to be a selective Type A picture: Type A empowered. That is, although Type As may have more challenge-seeking behavior, if accompanied by the classic Type A profile (hostility, anger, depression), the Type As tend to crack under the load.

    The solution: Type A classic (go-getter + perfectionism + success-driven) minus hostility = Type A empowered.

Q Is there an historical **gender** difference on coping?

■ In a recent report, researchers studied the calamities that beset the westward-bound settlers in 19th-century America. Most striking was the finding that nearly twice as many men died as women (57% vs 28%). Of those settlers who tried to snowshoe out of the mountains where they were stranded, all the men died and all the women survived. Possible reason: better insulation (body fat), plus less panic.

Q Stress and **nutrition**: what can be done?

■ A University of Alabama study found that rats subjected to stress had lower levels of the stress hormone cortisol when they were fed the human equivalent of several grams of Vitamin C a day. Cortisol can also suppress your immune system, which is why stress has been known to increase the risk of getting ill. Taking large daily doses of Vitamin C (over 2 grams/day) may also counteract that effect and help keep you healthy during times of stress. The study results also suggest that current governmental guidelines for Vitamin C intake (60 mg a day) may be too low.

Meanwhile, a recent Californian study found that alcohol empties your brain of chemicals that make you feel good – neurotransmitters such as dopamine, serotonin and gamma aminobutyric acid that affect your brain's pleasure pathways. The brain attempts to compensate by dramatically increasing corticotrophin-releasing factor, a stress chemical that leads to depression. This combination of decreased neurotransmitters and increased corticotrophin-releasing factor leaves your brain in a state of dependence – it wants more alcohol to get things back to normal.

So if you're under major stress, load up on Vitamin C – take the supplements periodically throughout the day, because your body flushes out excess Vitamin C every time you urinate. And lastly, go easy on the after-work drinks – they're not as relaxing as you thought.

Q. What is meant by "**nervous breakdown**," and what general warning symptoms can be perceived?

■ "Nervous breakdown" is a lay term, not an official diagnosis, so there's no specific definition and its meaning may vary. The general public seems to use it as a catch-all term to describe an acute emotional or psychological collapse.

Breathing and Smoking

Q What is the physiology of **nicotine**?

■ At lower blood levels, nicotine causes mild sedation and relaxation, which is precisely why most people use cigarettes during acute anxiety attacks. The sedative effect gives way to a stimulatory effect at higher dosages, thereby delaying the onset of sleep. The $T_{\frac{1}{2}}$ of nicotine is 2 hours. An average to heavy smoker sleeps between 30–60 minutes less than a non-smoker.

Q Does smoking directly affect my **blood pressure**?

■ In addition to thickening the blood, smoking cigarettes causes an explosion in BP due to a radical O_2 mismatch (abruptly decreasing O_2 availability combined with critical increases in demand during stressful moments). Try checking your BP during a cigarette smoke to see what the heart is witnessing. This is one of the reasons why cigarette smoking is responsible for 21% of all mortality from heart disease.

Q Is **passive smoking** (PS) dangerous?

■ Because of the toxins and carcinogens (*) in cigarette smoke – nitroamines ammonia, cyanhydric acid (used in gas chambers), acetone/toluene (solvents), methane (swamp gas), naphthalene, carbon monoxide (constituent of car exhaust fumes), phenol, DDT (insecticide), toluidine*, urethane*, dimethyl-nitrosamines*, naphthylamines*, pyrene*, polonium–210* (radioactive), cadmium* (a heavy metal found in car batteries), vinyl chloride* (a plastic) and benzopyrene* – passive smoking (PS) is associated with respiratory illnesses, asthma, and lung cancers (PS is responsible for over 3,000 deaths a year in the USA). Studies following smoking mothers' babies, showed a "dose-related increase" in hospitalizations (three times if mother smokes one pack per day), asthma (twofold increase), increased ear infections, incidences of sudden infant death syndrome and increased incidence of lung cancer as adults.

Q Do **smoke-free** policies work?

■ In a study based on a company with 15,000 employees who developed a no-smoking policy, 25% of smokers quit outright (peer pressure in reverse), there were 13% fewer medical visits for respiratory complaints and an annual saving of US$110,000. Such policies work for the people, whether smokers or non-smokers.

Body and Mind

Q I have heard that we use only 10% of the brain. What is happening to the **other 90%**?

■ The full answer is not yet clear, but one thing is certain: Nature, in her economical manner, does not make trivial decisions. She has bestowed upon us, in a relatively short time from an evolutionary point of view (10 million years), a massive cerebral cortex with limitless potential and capacity. For what function? Certainly not mere physical survival. In the book *Doors of Perceptions*, Huxley invites his readers to leave behind the noise of the marketplace of everyday life and use that brain capacity to expand the mind, build rooms in our soul for future refuge and develop our true potential as well as a greater understanding of life and each other. As James Joyce once wrote: "We are all in the gutter, except that some of us are looking at the stars."

Q Is **depression** more common in **heart attack patients**?

■ According to *Circulation*, the journal of the American Heart Association, depression and withdrawal are very common among heart attack patients. Depressed patients are approximately three times as likely to die when compared to non-depressed patients. The single most important factor in alleviating depression is strong social support, which may protect patients from the negative aspects of depression and improve their overall prognosis.

Q What is the relation between **smoking** and **aging**?

■ Both smoking and high BP accelerate the normal aging processes, accounting for 15% of the damaged abnormal brain tissue seen on MRI scans.[8] Behaviour in mid-life can make a difference in what faculties we have to enjoy later on.

Q **Stress** and **asthma**: what is the connection?

■ Studies have shown a clear causal relationship between anxiety, attack frequency, the medications required to control asthma, and asthma hospitalizations. Not only can stress trigger an asthmatic attack, it worsens the severity of the attack.

Q Does poorly controlled stress make us **stupid**?

■ A recent report, presented at the NeuroScience 2000 Conference, suggests that chronic releases of the stress hormone, cortisol, actually kill brain cells, an effect of chronic stress that is particularly evident in the memory centers. These hormones, glucocorticoids, also induce diabetes, high BP, high TG and colitis.

SELF-ASSESSMENT QUIZ

1 The only control I have in life is the way I react or respond to external pressure:

(a) True
(b) False

Hint: Freedom starts in the mind

2 Memory problems are a sign of:

(a) Serious mental problems
(b) Poor listening

(c) Lack of concentration

(d) Fate

Hint: Mind-control exercises (meditation and mantra) will help regain memory

3 The benefits of laughing are:

(a) Decreased BP

(b) Increased adrenaline

(c) Enhanced immune system

(d) Decreased oxygen to muscle

Hint: Humor is the best antidote to stress and life

4 The best time to practise meditation:

(a) am

(b) Lunchtime

(c) pm

Hint: As often as you need to center your mind

5 Mantra is strictly used for religious purposes:

(a) True

(b) False

Hint: Mantra is universal

6 After practicing alternative nostril breathing, I feel light-headed because:

(a) Oxygen has increased in my blood

(b) CO_2 has decreased in my blood

(c) Neither

Hint: Low CO_2 has that effect initially

7 You need a special place to do meditation:

(a) True

(b) False

8 If not taken care of, adrenaline can wake you up at night:

(a) True

(b) False

Hint: Mantra is universal

9 Deep breathing is time-consuming
- (a) True
- (b) False

Hint: Do it continually

10 Meditation can lower your blood pressure without medications:
- (a) True
- (d) False

Hint: Staying detached is good for the heart

11 How long do you need to meditate in the morning?
- (a) 5 minutes
- (b) 15 minutes
- (c) 30 minutes

Hint: As long as it takes to quiet the mind and smile

Answers

1 (b)	**5** (b)	**9** (b)
2 (b) & (c)	**6** (b)	**10** (a)
3 (a) & (c)	**7** (b)	**11** All
4 All	**8** (a)	

Notes

1 In his seminal book, *Zen Mind, Beginner's Mind* (Weatherhill Publishers, 1994), Shunryu Suzuki elaborates, "The mind of the beginner is empty, free of the habits of the expert, ready to accept, to doubt, and open to all the possibilities."

2 "Neuroendocrine and stress hormone change during mirthful laughter," *American Journal of Medical Science*, 1989, Dec.; 298 (6): 390–6.

3 An interpretation is offered by a learned student of the Upanishads, Eknath Easwaran: "First, we are neither body or mind; these simply make up the vehicle with which we travel through life. Second, there is a purpose to the mind. It is not supposed to lounge around emoting and desiring; its job is to guide the senses, pulling them up when they start to run after something pleasant instead of going where we want to go. And the intellect is not supposed to sit in an ivory tower and classify things that do not matter. Its job is to discriminate between preya ('that which is pleasant') and shreya ('that which is good'), choose wisely, and tell the mind what to do."

4 In a landmark study, 1,862 people completed a survey wherein they reported a market decrease in (1) hard liquor intake, (2) cigarette smoking and (3) lung abuse by mind-centering with meditation (Benson and Wallace, 1972).

5 People distracted by past events or future plans consisently miss present lessons while putting their lives and limbs at risk while driving automobiles.

6 From *Brihadaranyaka Upanishad*. See T. S. Eliot, *The Wasteland*: V What the Thunder Said.

7 Available on an excellent CD presentation by Times Music (India).

CHAPTER SEVEN

SPECIAL TOPICS

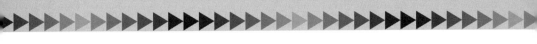

Using the advice contained in this chapter, Mr Timebomb could take care of the following health issues:

- low stamina (body fat)
- men's issues
- women's issues
- children's issues
- future trends

Stamina

There are four basic steps you can follow to achieve stamina and then retain it:

1 *Snack between meals*: out with the coffee break, in with the energy break: fresh or dried fruit and fresh water.

2 *Get high-octane fuel into the system*: eat only certain foods that are low in GI. *No fast foods*!

3 *Tune the body*: it's 3 pm, between meetings, you find yourself with 15 minutes and a lull in energy: use your desk or sink, and do 25 quick push-ups and 25 "crunches" (half sit-ups). If you have more time: the full 4-minute workout or the FIT program (get thee to a gym!).

4 *Oxygenate the brain*: find a quiet corner (office, taxi, toilet), close your eyes and push the "reset button": take ten deep breaths Visualize something peaceful, an evergreen forest or inland lake. Escape and smile!

Men's Issues

Q Does it matter how **fast** I eat?

■ Eating faster means later satiety and, hence, more calories which are associated with increased risk of a heart attack. Bolting the food also causes flatulence (from swallowed N_2).

Q What are the causes of **impotence**?

■ Approximately 40% of cases of penile dysfunction are the result of blood vessel disease. Other reasons include fatigue, prescription drugs, diabetes, stress, depression, drug dependency and alcohol dependency.

Q Are there any health implications of **impotence**?

■ In a recent study which reviewed the histories of 50 men with erectile dysfunction who had sought a prescription for Viagra (a drug to treat impotence), it was found that, although none had symptoms heart disease, 40% were found to have significant blockage and risk heart attacks.

Q How can I fight the discomfort of an **inflamed prostate** (prostatitis)?

■ Urologists have been having moderate success with prostatitis by eliminating spicy foods, caffeine (coffee, colas and chocolate) and alcohol.

Women's Issues

Q Are there differences between women and men for **heart attacks**?

■ Risk of death due to coronary artery disease (CAD) in women is roughly similar to that of men 10 years younger.
    Studies examining gender differences in heart attacks, found not only differences in the *type* of heart attack, but also found that among women less than 50 years of age the *rate of death* was twice that of men, due to higher complication rates.[1]

Q What about women and the **pill**?

■ The newer generations of oral contraceptives have an excellent risk/benefit ratio, except for women who also smoke.

Q What is the link between physical exercise and **breast cancer**?

■ According to researchers at the Salk Institute and USC, as little as three hours per week of exercise during her reproductive years could reduce the risk of breast cancer for a woman by 20–30%. After comparing more than 500 breast cancer patients with women without the disease, the researchers concluded that an average of four or more hours of physical activity per week gave a 60% risk reduction.

Q Is there any role for **Vitamin E** in the prevention of heart disease in menopausal women?

■ By eating foods high in Vitamin E (nuts, vegetable and fish oils, whole grains and wheat germ), post-menopausal women could reduce their risk for heart disease, according to a study presented to the American Heart Association in 2000.

Q **Future trends** for women's health?

■ Women may have different risk factors for heart disease. Researchers have found that a simple non-invasive test (Electron Beam Computed Tomography – EBCT), which measures calcium in the coronary artery, could better identify post-menopausal women at risk.

■ HRT + antioxidants Vitamin C + Vitamin E could be the right cocktail for improving insulin sensitivity, lowering plaque-inducing LDL cholesterol, and improving the overall risk profile for heart disease.

■ Soy protein: in soy products, there is a phytoestrogen called genistein, which may help in the fight against breast cancer, as evidenced by the lower incidence of breast cancer in Asian women where soy is a staple of the diet. The mechanism? The phytoestrogen in soy, by competing with estrogen for the estrogen receptor, lowers the estrogen level and increases the antioxidant capabilities to block free radical formation. Awaiting more research.

Q How often should a **mammogram** be done?

■ Annual screening mammography for women after the age of 40.

■ Clinical breast examinations by a health professional at least every three years beginning at age 20 and annually after age 40.

■ Monthly breast self-examination beginning by age 20.

■ Important exceptions to the above guidelines: women under age 40 with either a family history of breast cancer or other concerns about their personal risk should consult a trained medical professional about when to begin screening mammography.

Children's Issues

Q What are the risks for children who are **obese**?

■ Childhood obesity is a growing problem, associated with major medical and psychological implications for the children. Researchers found that young people with above average body fat (BF > 20%) during adolescence had greater insulin levels, BP and cholesterol in adulthood. 80% of obese children become obese adults. Moreover, if the fat is distributed around the waist (WHR > 0.85), the children had increased BP, TGs, cholesterol and decreased HDL, just like the adults.

   Attention to children does *not* mean unlimited sugar intake. Yes, spoil with encouragement, but don't ruin with sweets!

Q Why are **parents** not looking after their children's health better?

■ In a recent study, researchers interviewed 620 mothers of children aged 2–5 years of age. Of the 130 obese mothers, only 20% had an accurate perception of their obese children as being obese.

Premature Aging

Q What are feasible strategies against **premature aging**?

■ Eat slowly and with gusto.

■ Eat *less*: consuming 33% fewer calories can increase a rodent lifespan (less likely to get cancer) by 30% over more satiated animals. That is because, when satiated, animals secrete a protein called Insulin Growth Factor-1(IGF-1), which play an important function in premature aging and tumor growth.[2]

■ Develop conspiracies: exercise isn't the only way to stay young. Keeping close with your special someone may provide some of the same benefits. Research has shown that long-lasting, loving relationships provide long-lasting health benefits. In fact, studies have revealed that a successful marriage has a higher correlation with arterial youth than does low cholesterol. One way to improve your relationship this winter is to snuggle up after work and talk.

Future Trends for Health

The rising levels of obesity in children and adults are a dominant (and very worrying) feature when looking at future trends for overall health. Education on the standards for obesity need to be updated and customized; because of the smaller frames in East Asians, they misrepresent the drastic state of health affairs. If adopted, new standards would reveal the following picture:

■ In Malaysia: 20% of the population would be considered obese, instead of 6%.

■ In Taiwan: 16% of the population would be considered obese, instead of 4%.

■ In the Philippines: 13% of the population would be considered obese, instead of 3%.

We are increasingly looking to alternative models of health and medicine. In particular, the future trend appears to be towards those appraoches that are more holistic, effective and economical. Two examples include Indian (Ayurvedic) and Chinese (the Qi-centered approach).
Some facts about the Chinese model:

■ It has one of the oldest pharmacopoeia, started over 2,000 years ago with 365 plant, mineral and animal listings, and now topping over 12,000 listings.

■ According to the American Heart Association an extract of red yeast fermented on rice reduces cholesterol levels by 25%, reduces LDL by 33% and reduces TGs by 20%.

■ Westernized Chinese have been found to have thickening of the linings of their neck arteries (a sign of developing arteriosclerosis) – more than 20% thicker than those of villagers in China – pointing up the protective effects of the traditional Chinese diet, according to a study presented at the American Heart Association Scientific Sessions. Recommendations included:
  – more tofu (soy protein)
  – more green tea
  – less dairy products, less sugar, and less red meat
  – less deep frying, more steaming and stir-frying.

Notes

1 *New England Journal of Medicine*, 2000, July.

2 *Cancer Research*, 57: 4667.

EPILOGUE

BENEFITS FOR THE BUSINESS COMMUNITY

As seen throughout the discussion in this book, the business community, perhaps more than any other subset of the world's population, is particularly susceptible to heart disease, strokes, diabetes, stress-related disorders, depression and marital conflict. Our research with more than 30,000 managers while based at INSEAD since 1988 indicates that this situation need *not* be so. We have innovated many tools to be made available to the modern manager so they can avoid the hazards of their profession.

This work is based not merely upon the published clinical research findings of eminent scientists worldwide, but also upon our own research while teaching at INSEAD and Stanford University.

Our Research

When working with managers, we discovered that it isn't mere intensity that yields results in relation to the 6Ws of health and sanity, it is focus. That is, instead of attempting the impossible of completely changing their lifestyles, we simply supervised the development of a feasible and effective Health Action Plan for each manager. One test group in particular, we called Mr Timebomb, as their health and sanity were in a very precarious position. These managers had failed *every* regimen, *every* fad diet, *every* stress management program, *every* encouragement. In Table E.1 you can see that their average actual age was 47.6 years of age but they had an average health age of 65.2 years of age, due to all the risk factors

In just 6 months of doing some of the 6Ws they completely and easily transformed their lives and health profile

present. This amounts to a cumulative loss of productive years among these 100 Mr Timebombs of 1,760 years!

We proved that these people were not meant to be "casualties of the profession": in just 6 months of doing some of the 6Ws they completely and easily transformed their lives and health profile (see Table E.1).

TABLE E.1 *100 Timebomb managers: baseline and after six months*

Health parameters	Ideal ranges	Baseline	+ 6 months
Actual age (AA)		47.6	48.2
Health age (HA)		65.2	46.3
Productive years	HA–AA X 100	Lost = 1,760 years	Regained = 1,760 + years
Blood pressure	< 135/85	155/95	135/82
Body fat	Men < 20%, Women < 23%	28	22
Kg as fat		32	21
Activity survey	Survey score > 8/10	4.5	6.5
Nutrition survey	Survey score > 8/10	5.6	8.2
Stress survey	Survey score > 8/10	4.6	7.8
Waist-to-hip ratio	< 0.85	1.13	0.96
Cardio-fitness	< 86–93 beats	145	102
Resting heart rate	< 68	78	64
Press-ups	> 20	7	30
Curl-ups	> 65	12	55
Squats	> 45	13	45
Laboratory analysis	**Ideal ranges**	**Baseline**	**+ 6 months**
Total cholesterol (TC)	< 2.0 grams/liter	2.90	2.10
HDL cholesterol	> 0.50 grams/liter	0.30	0.50

Laboratory analysis	Ideal ranges	Baseline	+ 6 months
TC:HDL ratio	< 4	9.7	4.2
LDL cholesterol	< 1.30 grams/liter	2.08	1.26
VLDL cholesterol	< 0.30 grams/liter	0.52	0.24
Triglycerides (TGs)	< 1.40 grams/liter	2.60	1.20
TG:HDL ratio	< 2	8.67	2.40
Fasting blood sugar (FBS)	0.70 –1.20 grams/liter	2.10	1.10

Accounting for Time

Say you find about 20 minutes a day, every day. That's a 10-minute walk after your heaviest meal, one 4-minute workout, and a 6-minute meditation session every morning. That is equal to 7,300 minutes, – a *total* yearly investment of 5.1 days for the benefit of your health and sanity. For those five days of investment, your health age will improve from 42 years to 66 years, a net gain of 24 years!

Reflect for a moment. Given the frenzied state of the world today, *somebody* should. Life is accelerating at an ever-increasing speed. Nobody even knows how to wait anymore. Consider your time disposition. How much time do you spend happy and fulfilled? In fact, by the time we reach 60 years of age (retirement), we have engaged in:

- **sleep** (22 years)
- **work** (20 years)
- **eating** (eight years)
- **commuting** (five years, mostly locked in traffic)
- six years of **daily routines** (180 days looking in the mirror, 545 days for women)
- **good news:** 15 years left for projects *after* retirement.

Time waits for no one! Know where your time is going before it's all frittered away. Use the Health Action Plans below, designed for the busy fast-tracker who wants to stay out of the clinic and in the fast track as long as possible. *Bon courage!*

Health Action Plan (Stage I)

You are in Stage I if: you smoke > 20 cigarettes a day, or your BP is > 160/100, or your BF > 25%, or LDL > 1.60 g/l, or TG/HDL > 5, or CF > 130 beats.

M	T	W	Th	F	Sa	Su
4' WO (Stage I)	4' WO (Stage I)	4' WO (Stage I)	4' WO (Stage I)	4' WO (Stage I)	4' WO (Stage I)	Rest
Low GI + 15' walk	Low GI + 15' walk	Low GI + 15' walk	Low GI + 15' walk	Low GI + 15' walk	Low GI + 15' walk	High GI+ 45' walk
Snack: fruits + nuts, H_2O between meals	Snack: fruits + nuts, H_2O between meals	Snack: fruits + nuts, H_2O between meals	Snack: fruits + nuts, H_2O between meals	Snack: fruits + nuts, H_2O between meals	Snack: fruits + nuts, H_2O between meals	Snack: fruits + nuts, H_2O between meals
Red wine with dinner + PMR	Red wine with dinner + PMR	Red wine with dinner + PMR	Red wine with dinner + PMR	Red wine with dinner + PMR	Red wine with dinner + PMR	Red wine with dinner + PMR

Key

1 4' WO = 4-minute workout (see Chapter 4, p. 103).
2 GI = Glycemic Index (see Chapter 1, p. 24).
3 PMR = Progressive muscular relaxation (see p. 87).

Measuring fat (see p. 17) in four weeks: expect to have lost up to 5% body fat. This has worked for other Stage I fast-trackers; it will work well for you within 6–8 weeks.

Health Action Plan (Stage II)

You are in Stage II if: you smoke < 20 cigarettes a day, or your BP is between 140/90–160/100, or LDL is 1.30–1.60 g/l, or TG/HDL is 3–5, or your BF is between 20–25%, or CF > 100–130 beats.

M	T	W	Th	F	Sa	Su
4' WO (Stage II) + AO	4' WO (Stage II) + AO	FIT 30 30 minutes	4' WO (Stage II) + AO	4' WO (Stage II) + AO	4' WO (Stage II) + AO	FIT 30 minutes
Low GI +15' walk	Low GI +15' walk	High GI +15' walk	Low GI +15' walk	Low GI +15' walk	Low GI +15' walk	High GI +15' walk
Snack: fruits + nuts, H_2O between meals	Snack: fruits + nuts, H_2O between meals	Snack: fruits + nuts, H_2O between meals	Snack: fruits + nuts, H_2O between meals	Snack: fruits + nuts, H_2O between meals	Snack: fruits + nuts, H_2O between meals	Snack: fruits + nuts, H_2O between meals
Red wine with dinner + meditation	Red wine with dinner + meditation	Red wine with dinner + meditation	Red wine with dinner + meditation	Red wine with dinner + meditation	Red wine with dinner + meditation	Red wine with dinner + meditation

Key

1 4' WO = 4-minute workout (see Chapter 4, p. 106).

3 AO = Antioxidant treatment (see Chapter 3, p. 78).

4 GI = Glycemic Index (see Chapter 1, p. 24).

5 FIT : Aerobic cardio-fitness : 2 X / week for 30 minutes (see Chapter 4, p. 115).

Measuring fat (see p. 17) in four weeks: expect to have lost up to 5% body fat. This has worked for other Stage II fast-trackers; it will work well for you.

Health Action Plan (Stage III)

You are in Stage III if: you don't smoke, and your BP < 140/90, and LDL < 1.30 g/l, and TG/HDL < 3, and BF < 20%, and CF < 100 beats.

M	T	W	Th	F	Sa	Su
4' WO (Stage III) + DB + AO	FIT for 45 minutes	4' WO (Stage III) + DB + AO	FIT for 45 minutes	4' WO (Stage III) + DB + AO	4' WO (Stage III) + DB + AO	FIT for 45 minutes
Low GI + 15' walk	High GI	Low GI + 15' walk	High GI	Low GI + 15' walk	Low GI + 15' walk	High GI
Snack: fruits + nuts, H_2O between meals	Snack: fruits + nuts, H_2O between meals	Snack: fruits + nuts, H_2O between meals	Snack: fruits + nuts, H_2O between meals	Snack: fruits + nuts, H_2O between meals	Snack: fruits + nuts, H_2O between meals	Snack: fruits + nuts, H_2O between meals
Red wine with dinner + meditation or PMR or DB	Red wine with dinner + meditation or PMR or DB	Red wine with dinner + meditation or PMR or DB	Red wine with dinner + meditation or PMR or DB	Red wine with dinner + meditation or PMR or DB	Red wine with dinner + meditation or PMR or DB	Red wine with dinner + meditation or PMR or DB

Key

1 4' WO = 4-minute workout (see Chapter 4, p. 109).

2 DB = Deep breathing (see Chapter 6, p. 184).

3 AO = Antioxidant treatment (see Chapter 3, p. 78).

4 GI = Glycemic Index (see Chapter 1, p. 24).

5 FIT : Aerobic cardio-fitness : 3 X / week for 45 minutes (see Chapter 4, p. 115).

Measuring fat (see p. 17) in four weeks: expect to have lost up to 5% body fat. This has worked for other Stage III fast-trackers.

Objectives-oriented Nutrition

We need different forms of nutrition for our differing needs and desires. For example, the following advice applies when we need:

1 Nutrition for *energy* (battling fatigue):

- go for a 15-minute brisk walk after lunch;
- for high stamina, avoid alcohol at lunchtime;
- snack intelligently between meals (to avoid low blood sugar): fruit and nuts ideal;
- diminish your coffee intake;
- drink 2–3 liters fresh water a day (between meals!) or the equivalent: fruits, soups or vegetables.

2 Nutrition for effective and lasting *weight control*:

- eat foods with a low Glycemic Index;
- go for a 15-minute brisk walk after lunch;
- eat a light dinner and walk briskly afterwards;
- snack between meals (to control hunger): fruit is ideal;
- drink two glasses of water just before lunch and dinner.

3 Nutrition for *optimal health:*

- stay "regular" with fiber and Vitamin C: fruits and vegetables;
- prefer fish and skinless chicken to red meats;
- eat foods as close as possible to their natural raw state: avoid deep-fried foods!;
- every month, do a fruit fast (at home): just juices and fresh fruits all day to clean out all digestive residue in the gut;
- drink 2–3 liters fresh water a day (between meals!) or the equivalent: fruits, soups or vegetables.

How Did We Do It?

We *listened* to the more than 30,000 managers who participated in the Health Management Program, either at INSEAD or within their corporations. Several realities emerged, with some consistency, from this vast pool of managers from all over the world:

- You need to gain control of your life: maintain the health of the body (the horse) by keeping the mind active (the rider).
- You can measure your overall health and body fat with a tape measure.
- Critical risk factors are easy to control: body fat, blood pressure, stress management, smoking, activity level and so on.
- Be scientific! Adopt an engineering mindset: you must experiment with the available tools.
- *You* can decide, armed with the right tools, when you peak. Shoot for 70 years of age: a few million in the bank, children through university, spouse in good health. These are truly the Golden Years!

Here are some of the *tools* that we innovated while listening to the managers:

- **The 6Ws to peak health**: Walking, Water, Wine, Workout, Worrying effectively and Wind. The beauty of this Lazy Person's Program is that, using these ancient tools from the world's cultures, which respect your DNA, you can adapt the 6Ws to optimize health and fitness, according to your particular culture, at your pace, and without giving up much (remember: compensation works better than deprivation!).
- **Health Management Program (HMP)**: = one day seminar.
- **The Game**: a competitive game sponsored by the McGannon Institute of Practice Health (MIPH).
- **Urban Warrior's Interactive Network (UWIN)**: each and every participant receives an internet access code for him/herself, as well as one for their partner (http://mcgannon.insead.fr/HMP/).
- **Passport Edition**: plastic passport card that is a distillate of the course, used a reference card and bookmark.

Finally, to end on a positive note, remember what has been said at several points in this book and what, indeed, our research has confirmed – a solid work–life balance is possible.

Making Contact

There are several ways to avail oneself of the above tools:

1 By e-mail:

At the McGannon Institute of Proactive Health (MIPH):

- McGannoninstitute@compuserve.com

At INSEAD:

- Michael.McGannon@insead.edu

2 By telephone or fax:

At MIPH:

- (331) 64310421 (telephone)
- (331) 64310422 (fax)

At INSEAD:

- (331) 60724161 (telephone)

3 By post:

- c/o McGannon Institute of Proactive Health

  25 rue de Flagy
  77940 Thoury-Ferrottes
  France

- c/o INSEAD

  Blvd de Constance

  77350 Fontainebleau

  France

►►► Index

▶▶▶ *Acclaim for this book*

The McGannons have a know-how and contagious enthusiasm that has changed my life. Thousands of participants at INSEAD have greatly appreciated Dr. McGannon's first book, *The Urban Warrior's Book of Solutions*, and this, their second book, is a beautiful marriage between American science and French savoir vivre.

PROFESSOR JEAN-CLAUDE LARRÉCHÉ, INSEAD

The McGannon Institute has an extremely practical and user friendly health care review and management programme. In the short time of a day one can learn key health tracking and control tools and walk away with simple techniques to stay fit. *Highly* recommended.

MR. ANALJIT SINGH, CHAIRMAN, MAX INDIA LIMITED

With health, everything is possible – it truly is. This book is an inspirational example of how yoou can take charge of your well-being. The suggestions are practical and grounded in the reality of what can be achieved in the life of a hard-driven executive in today's competitive marketplace.

MR. RAVI BHOOTHALINGAM, PRESIDENT, THE OBEROI GROUP, DELHI, INDIA

Rarely has one come across a Health Management Program which can indeed be part of day-to-day management practices as are detailed here. Presented in this book are extremely simple, practical and yet invaluable tools critical to preserving ththe most important part of life: i.e. health. I wish this could be mandated in the corporate world.

MR. ASHWANI WINDLASS, CHAIRMAN, ARGUS INFRASTRUCTURE LTD

The Health Management Program laid out here must be an essential interlude in the overtly lopsided lifestyle of the busy business executive. It not only provides a jolting reminder that all is not necessarily well, but shows a very practical way forward towards a 'balanced' approach to life. Companies should consider mandating this program for all employees. Juliette and Mike deserve kudos for their pioneering approach which puts 'good health' within the grasp of everyone!

MR. DALJIT SINGH, EXECUTIVE DIRECTOR, ICI INDIA LIMITED

People are our firm's *core asset* and their health is a matter of great concern for us. Dr. and Mrs. McGannon's program allows us to ensure that our people are proactive in managing their health and the many pressures facing them in today's business environment. The program is central to the culture and values of our firm. Commitment to the program's action points ensures a better quality of life. Our people really enjoy it and have benefited significantly from it.

PAUL HENNESSY, VALUES PARTNER, PRICEWATERHOUSECOOPERS, IRELAND

Juliette and Michael give herein very practical advice on how to achieve worklife balance which is crucial to our managers today. His holistic approach to the individual, looking at the effects of diet, exercise and stress on their health and stamina is both delivered and received with great enthusiasm. The Health Management Program is one of the most essential and enjoyable programs we run and has become a core program in our Learning and Education Calendar of events.

SHEILA CURTIN, LEARNING AND EDUCATION LEADER, PwC, IRELAND

In their corporate training program, Mike and Juliette show that all individuals can and should achieve emotional, intellectual and spiritual fulfillment, as well as abolishing negative and unproductive habits. Their right livelihood mantra' practicing, which is an eminently easy and do-able tool, gives us an opportunity to enjoy a healthy, and vigorous lifestyle.

MR. AMITABH HAJELA, HEAD, LEADERSHIP RESOURCING,
GENERAL ELECTRIC CAPITAL, INDIA

Work, travel and pressure – all increasing for today's busy executives. The McGannons' clear, straightforward and practical approach in their Health Management Program for executives is indispensable in keeping our work and personal lives in balance, is excellent and easy, in minutes a day. It's made a substantial impact on my ability to be healthy, productive and happy!

MR. MARK LANGHAMMER, SENIOR VICE PRESIDENT,
ECONOMIST INTELLIGENCE UNIT, ASIA PACIFIC

In 1971, it was discovered during a routine medical that my triglyceride levels were high – very high. At the time knowledge of triglycerides was rudimentary, and I underwent a series of tests, medications and diet changes designed to reduce the high level. Nothing worked. Over the last 30 years, no matter what I've tried, and no matter the advice from my various doctors, I was unable to reduce the triglyceride levels from around 2.50–3.00 against a desirable level of 0.12–1.71.

In June 2000, I participated in Dr. McGannon's Health Management Plan. At the time he claimed that he knew exactly why my triglycerides were high, and the action required to reduce them. Although sceptical, I followed his advice rigorously for four months and repeated the blood tests. To my (and my doctor's) astonishment, my triglyceride levels were down to 1.44, well within the accepted desirable level for the first time ever. I would therefore encourage anyone who values their health, and is keen to correct any imbalances, to listen to Dr. Michael McGannon, and follow his advice. All it takes is some minor adjustments to lifestyle habits, but the benefits are enormous. It's all here!

MR. JIM McCALLUM, PwC, LONDON

Good for body, mind and our team spirit. Michael and Juliette McGannon's down-to-earth and easy to understand communication style complemented by his great visual displays, made an immediate and lasting impression. As a result we all adjusted our lifestyles and still practice much of what he taught us. Great for all!

MR. FRITZ HORLACHER, PRESIDENT, ZUELLIG PHARMA, HONG KONG